HOLD THE POWER

Isometric Hold Training

Kevin B. DiBacco

FOREWORD

PROFESSIONAL ENDORSEMENTS

Isometric strength training is one of the most underrated, and sometimes forgotten, strategies for building strength. Isometric conditioning of the muscles enjoys a great safety profile, generally with minimal risk for injury. Kevin has mastered the science of isometric conditioning and has put together programs that safely and effectively build quality muscle.

Dr. Val Fiott
ACE-Certified Health Coach and Personal Trainer
Subject Matter Expert for the American Council on Exercise
drval.perfectpersonaltraining.com

_____

I came across this wonderful book by Kevin. Isometric exercise has changed the way I work out, and it has helped me build up muscle without the wear and tear of traditional weight-lifting exercises. "Kevin has explained the exercise programs in simple words, and I would highly recommend this book to anyone who wants to know more about isometric training."

Dr. Fatima Tanveer
MBBS, M.D., ECFMG certified, Internal Medicine. MD Pakistan, Physician and International Medical Research Health, Medical & Lifestyle writer, South Asia.

DISCLAIMER

No part of this publication may be reproduced in any form or by any means, including printing, scanning, photocopying, or otherwise without the prior written permission of the copyright holder. The author has tried to present information that is as correct and concrete as possible. The author is not a medical doctor and does not write in any medical capacity. All medical decisions should be made under the guidance and care of your primary physician. The author will not be held liable for any injury or loss that is incurred to the reader through the application of any of the information here contained in this book. The author makes it clear that the medical field is fast evolving with newer studies being done continuously, therefore the information in this book is only a researched collaboration of accurate information at the time of writing. With the ever-changing nature of the subjects included, the author hopes that the reader will be able to appreciate the content that has been covered in this book. While all attempts have been made to verify each piece of information provided in this publication, the author assumes no responsibility for any error, omission, or contrary interpretation of the subject matter present in this book. Please note that any help or advice given hereof is not a substitution for licensed medical advice. The reader accepts responsibility in the use of any information and takes advice given in this book at their own risk. If the reader is under medication supervision or has had complications with health-related risks, consult your primary care physician as soon as possible before taking any advice given in this book.

"The information and advice contained in this book are based upon the research and the personal and professional experiences of the author. They are not intended as a substitute for consulting with a healthcare professional. The publisher and author are not responsible for any adverse effects or consequences resulting from the use of any of the suggestions, preparations, or procedures discussed in this book. All matters pertaining to your physical health should be supervised by a healthcare professional."

TABLE OF CONTENTS

Thank you to my biggest fans and my motivator, Rachel. A big thanks to my publisher, my cheerleader and my friend Andrea Bibby at Urban Viking Books for believing in my story.

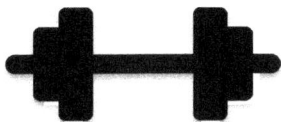

Kevin understands adversity and the temptation to quit better than most. His life has been a testament to the power of perseverance despite severe hardship. Now he shares his story and tools to inspire others to get off the mat when knocked down by life.

Kevin's health struggles began early, needing major surgery at just 16 years old. In his 20s and 30s, he endured 6 knee operations, 2 back surgeries including spinal fusion, 2 hip replacements, and treatment for an aggressive brain tumor. Enduring over 10 major medical procedures would be enough to make anyone want to give up. Even as he was writing this, Kevin was struck by Covid-19. As if that was not another setback, Kevin developed Pneumonia and spend the spring of 2022 and the summer of 2023 having to get daily nebulizer treatments. Once again, his theories were put to the test. Once again, they worked!

But Kevin refused to see himself as a victim of circumstance. Through each diagnosis and rehabilitation, he consciously worked to reframe adversity as an opportunity for growth. Instead of sadly ruminating on limitations, he focused positively on each small win - standing, walking, climbing stairs - during recovery. He visualized himself healed and happy, against all odds.

Kevin leaned on his deep faith and the support of loved ones during the darkest times. When fear or hopelessness crept in, he prayed for the strength to take the next step forward. He turned to uplifting books and sayings for encouragement. Slowly but surely, he reclaimed his active lifestyle step by step.

Through his journey, Kevin realized firsthand the power of mindset to determine one's experience of life. He discovered that by controlling his inner world - his thoughts, beliefs, visualizations - he could transform his outer reality. Now he hopes to share these lessons with others facing major life challenges.

Kevin's book recounts his medical battles, along with the techniques he used to stay grounded in positivity. He provides exercises to overcome negative self-talk, face fears, and visualize desired outcomes. Kevin believes we can all learn to reframe difficulties as growth opportunities. Wherever we feel like quitting, he urges us to proclaim, "I will keep going!"

Kevin's dramatic story provides living proof that, no matter what knocks us down, we can choose to get back up. We all have access to inner reserves of strength to endure the unendurable. Kevin hopes his book will inspire others to fight major life battles to find their power to keep progressing. By committing to personal growth, we can overcome any obstacle, including those within our own mind.

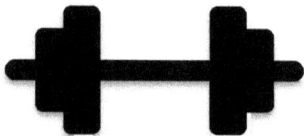

So, who am I? I'm a 60 something artist/writer that has lived at least 3 lives. As an athlete, as a filmmaker, and now as an author.

I have been a competitive powerlifter, semi pro baseball player, semi pro Softball player, played football, boxed and even tried tennis. I have been an athlete all my life. I did all that while pursuing my career as a television commercial producer and then professional filmmaker. Into my thirties injuries and surgeries slowed me down. Baseball, softball, football all took a back seat to weight training and powerlifting. For 30 years, I continued in the gym and competed in a few PUSH/ PULL competitions. It was around 1993 when I set an all-time bench press record for myself in the over 30 class, with a bench press of 515.

I moved around for my television career. It was in 2018 after fourteen years off from training, back surgery, brain surgery and double hip surgery that made me worry that I may never be in shape again. After spending more than half my life in the gym, the thought of never going back to workout just did not sit well with me. I decided that I would customize a program of Isometrics, resistance bands and dumbbells to see if I could rehab my hips, back, knee and my entire body. I must work muscles now that were severely compromised. I had to find a way to train injured body parts without re-injuring myself. I knew powerlifting was out. I couldn't even carry one forty-five-pound plate. Gone are the days of my impressive 515-pound bench press. I did my homework. While home recovering after hip surgery, I started reading the package my orthopedic surgeon gave me. All my exercises were Isometric type of physical therapy. I began to think, what if you can get strength back in your hip with Isometrics why not your back, shoulders, arms and chest? I read just about every book on Isometric training and especially Isometric holds. I still own all the books. There were about a dozen really good books going back to the 1900's. I trained with conventional weights for so long, I knew all my old exercises could be customized to be isometric movements. I started very slowly. My first goal was to learn how to walk on new hips with a lifelong back problem and nerve damage. It took months. I kept detailed notes, used bands instead of weights, and bought a total gym. I finally started to see progress. I lost 75 pounds from the years of whoopie pies and ice cream. Built a new diet. Eliminated sugar, dairy and started to feel like I had something here. I lost weight, lowered my a1c, blood pressure, heart rate, I was 25 again internally. The result of those years of experiments was my first book 'Hysometrics'. I had much more to share and one of the most important workout techniques there is, the Isometric Hold or to be more exact the **'OVERCOMING ISOMETRIC HOLD'.** I'm covering that here.

I hope you enjoy it. The fact is that I'm not just a guy that wrote a book about fitness, like thousands do. I authored a book on what I did to recover from severe injury and surgeries. How I was able to get mobile, strong and lose weight at the same time. It's not just a book, it's an in-depth journal on what got me back into shape when I thought all was lost. If I can do it with my bionic body, I KNOW you can too! Start slow, be patient and NEVER GIVE UP. You are much stronger than you think. No one is going to come to you if you want a healthy life pain free and normally you must build muscle strength. Muscle strength doesn't mean that you have to look like an NFL lineman. When I talk about muscle strength, I am talking about functional strength that you use every day. At work, gardening, shopping, etc. We all need muscle strength to live our normal lives. You can build muscle strength at any age from 18 or 80. This is a great start!

Kevin

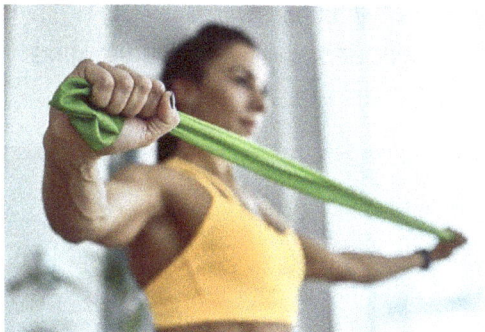

WHAT EXACTLY IS AN ISOMETRIC HOLD?

EVERYONE has seen an Isometric hold sometime in their life, rehabbing an injury, In the movies or just working out old muscles. Isometric holds have been around for years. The Military and Orthopedic doctors still use them today! They are also a great way to get into shape if you don't have the time or equipment. In this Book I cover One of the two Isometric HOLD TECHNIQUES, called the 'OVERCOMING ISOMETRIC HOLD'.

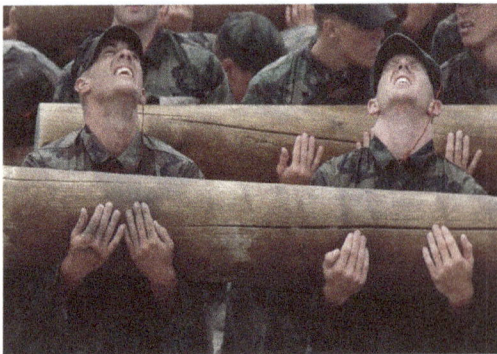

The log carry, also known as the log PT (physical training), is a common exercise performed in military training.
The log carry is often included in military training for several reasons:

Functional Fitness: The military aims to develop functional fitness, which means training the body to perform real-world tasks effectively. Carrying heavy loads, such as logs or equipment, is a common requirement in military operations. The log carry helps soldiers build strength and endurance specific to these demands.

Teamwork and Camaraderie: Military training emphasizes teamwork and cohesion among soldiers. The log carry is often performed as a team exercise, where a group of individuals carries a heavy log together. This fosters teamwork, communication, and a sense of camaraderie among the trainees.

Mental Resilience: The log carry can be physically demanding, requiring mental toughness and resilience to push through fatigue and discomfort. By incorporating exercises like the log carry, military training aims to develop mental fortitude, discipline, and the ability to persevere in challenging situations.

The log carry is not strictly classified as an isometric hold exercise. Isometric hold exercises involve static muscle contractions without joint movement, such as holding a plank position. In contrast, the log carry involves dynamic movements as soldiers walk or run while carrying the log. I would call it a 'yielding isometric exercise'. Similar to holding a bar, sandbag or plate in one position. You still have some movement in the joint.

Isometric Holds, also known as Isometric Exercise, is a method of resistance training that involves pushing or pulling against an immovable or unyielding object, such as an overloaded bar in a power rack or a locked exercise machine. This is different from yielding isometric exercises, where the weight is held motionless against gravity or the tension of a spring, resistance band or even weight bar.

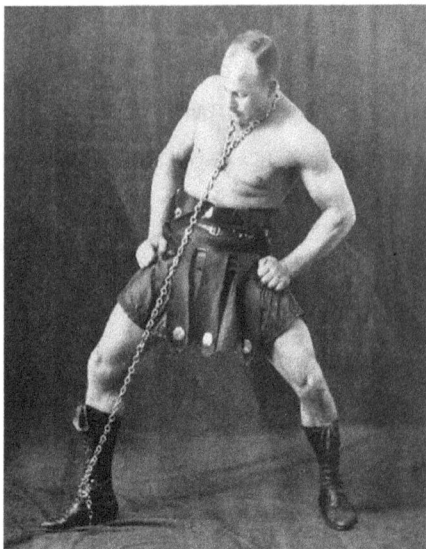

The earliest known proponents of isometric training was Alexander Zass, a Russian strongman and physical culture expert who lived from 1888 to 1962. Zass developed a type of isometric exercise known as "self-resistance," which involved contracting one's own muscles against each other to create resistance without the use of weights or other equipment.

Born in 1888 in Lithuania (then part of the Russian Empire), Zass developed an interest in physical strength from a youthful age. He trained in various physical disciplines, including wrestling, weightlifting, and bodybuilding. During World War I, Zass served in the Russian army and was taken as a prisoner of war by the Austro-Hungarian forces.

While in captivity, Zass used his physical abilities to his advantage. He devised a training routine that involved isometric exercises, where he would exert force against immovable objects, such as chains and bars. This form of training helped him maintain his strength despite the lack of conventional weights.

After his release from captivity, Zass embarked on a career as a strongman and circus performer. He amazed audiences with his incredible feats of strength, which included bending iron bars, lifting heavy weights, and even carrying horses on his back.

Zass is also credited with popularizing the concept of isometric exercise and promoting its benefits. He published a book titled "The Amazing Samson" in 1924, in which he described his training methods and shared his experiences.

While Alexander Zass may not be as widely recognized as some other strongmen of his time, his innovative approach to training and his remarkable displays of strength left a lasting impact on the world of physical fitness.

Alexander Zass utilized isometric exercises as a fundamental part of his training regimen. Isometric exercises involve exerting force against an immovable object or maintaining a static position against resistance, without any joint movement. Zass believed that isometric exercises were crucial for building strength and developing a powerful physique.

During his time as a prisoner of war, Zass had limited access to traditional weights and exercise equipment. To maintain his strength, he devised a training method centered around isometric exercises. He would find objects such as chains, bars, or tree branches and push, pull, or twist against them with maximal effort, holding the position for a certain duration.

By performing isometric exercises, Zass aimed to develop strong tendons, ligaments, and connective tissues, which he believed were essential for overall strength and injury prevention. These exercises allowed him to work his muscles without relying on external resistance or weights.

His isometric training routine involved a wide range of exercises targeting various muscle groups. He would perform pushing exercises like pushing against walls, pulling exercises like pulling on ropes or chains, and twisting exercises like twisting thick bars or chains. Additionally, he would incorporate squeezing exercises by gripping objects with maximal force.

By employing isometric exercises in his training, Zass was able to maintain and even enhance his strength despite his limited training environment. His innovative use of isometrics helped him develop remarkable feats of strength and establish himself as a notable figure in the world of physical fitness.

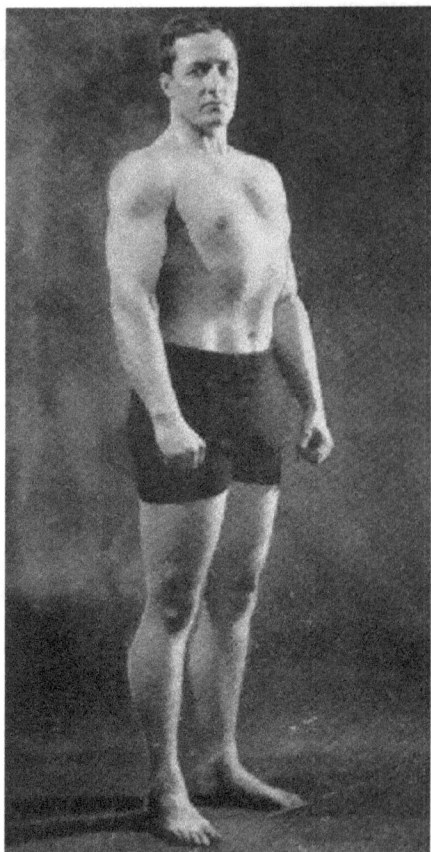

30

Another early advocate of isometric training was Bob Hoffman, the founder of the York Barbell Company and a pioneer of modern strength training. Hoffman began incorporating isometric exercises into his training routines in the 1940s, and his influence helped to popularize the concept among athletes and fitness enthusiasts.

Since then, isometric training has been used in a wide variety of contexts, including physical therapy, rehabilitation, and athletic training.

'Unlike traditional overcoming isometric methods, which involves multiple maximum effort contractions lasting a few seconds with varying rest periods in between, Isometric Holds involves a single continuous repetition of increasing intensity.

(The BEST PART is that Isometric holds can be a fantastic way to improve your strength and endurance, by using an eight-dollar strap, rope, or pet leash.)

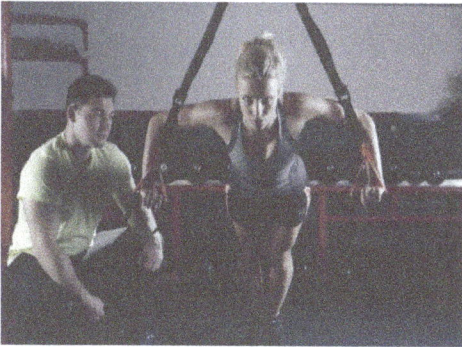

TWO TYPES OF ISOMETRICS

Yielding Isometrics:

Yielding isometrics are exercises in which the muscles are contracted to maintain a fixed position for a certain amount of time. In this type of isometric exercise, the muscle fibers are activated and the muscle contracts, but there is no actual movement of the joint.

Yielding isometric exercises can be performed by holding a static position against resistance for a set period of time. Examples of yielding isometric exercises include planks, wall sits, and static lunges.

In yielding isometrics, the goal is to keep a fixed position, typically for a few seconds to a few minutes, while resisting an external force. **By holding the position, the muscle is working against the resistance**, which creates tension in the muscle fibers. Over time, this tension can lead to increased strength, endurance, and overall muscular control.

One of the benefits of yielding isometric exercises is that they can be performed with little to no equipment, making them an accessible option for people who may not have access to a gym or other exercise equipment. Additionally, they are low impact, which means they are less likely to cause joint pain or injury compared to exercises that involve jumping or running.

OVERCOMING ISOMETRICS

Overcoming isometrics are exercises in which the muscles are contracted to generate maximal force against an immovable object or resistance. (the KEY DIFFERENCE is that the **weight or OBJECT is attached and immovable**). In this type of isometric exercise, the muscle fibers are activated and the muscle contracts, but there is no actual movement of the joint.

Overcoming isometric exercises can be performed by pushing against a wall, pulling on a door frame, or holding a heavy object that cannot be moved like a tree or jungle gym or even a car. In this type of isometric exercise, the goal is to generate maximum force against the immovable object or resistance for a brief period of time.

Overcoming isometrics are typically used to improve explosive power and the ability to generate maximal force. By generating maximal force against an immovable object or resistance, the muscle fibers are activated and the muscle contracts, which can lead to increased strength and power over time.

One of the benefits of overcoming isometric exercises is that they can be performed with little to no equipment, making them an accessible option for people who may not have access to a gym or other exercise equipment. Additionally, they can be an effective way to improve muscular strength and power without putting excessive stress on the joints.

Both yielding isometrics and overcoming isometrics can be effective for building strength, stability, and endurance in the muscles being worked. When incorporating isometric exercises into a workout routine, it's important to use proper form and to gradually increase the difficulty of the exercises over time to avoid injury and maximize the benefits.

HYSOMETRICS

Hysometrics is a program I developed after 40 years of Powerlifting.

Hysometrics which is basically a combination of Isometrics and dynamic exercises with weights, Iso-Bow or Bands. Done as a superset, back-to-back within your workout.

The Idea for Hysometrics is to utilize the BEST of both worlds. The Strength training of ISOMETRICS with the Muscle building and toning of Bands/Weights/Reps. Look for my book HYSOMETRICS!

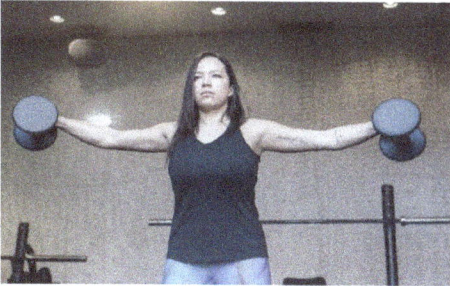

Compared to the rest-pause method, Isometric Holds offers increased safety and metabolic and cardiovascular conditioning. Gradually increasing force over a longer period of time reduces the risk of muscle strain, joint injury, or aggravating an existing injury. Fatiguing the target muscles with moderate and near-maximum effort phases reduces the level of force they can produce during the final maximum effort phase, allowing for an all-out effort with less risk of injury.

However, the force and tension in the muscle are still higher than during a dynamic set of similar duration.

Isometric Holds are a highly effective form of exercise that is widely regarded as one of the safest ways to work out, provided that it is performed correctly. One of the key benefits of this type of exercise is that it provides you with complete control over the force encountered during the workout, which means that you can stop at any time without having to worry about dropping weights or transferring weight to a different position.

Additionally, **Isometric Holds can be highly beneficial for individuals with a variety of joint and spine conditions**, as well as those with neurological disorders or motor control problems.

Many trainers and fitness enthusiasts have been using Isometric Holds for years, either on specialized machines designed for this purpose or by using power racks and safety bars. More recently, the UXS bodyweight multi-exercise station and straps have become popular tools for performing Isometric Hold exercises. By holding a static position, an Isometric Hold has enabled many individuals to perform exercises that previously caused them joint irritation or pain when performed dynamically.

However, there are a few disadvantages to using Isometric Holds as a form of exercise. One of the biggest challenges is that, without specialized equipment capable of measuring force input, it can be challenging to quantify your performance and progress over time. When you are contracting isometrically against an immobile object, there is no weight, repetitions, only a hold time to measure, count, or record. As a result, if you want to be able to evaluate your progress over time, it is necessary to occasionally perform a few test exercises for the major muscle groups using either dynamic reps (weight x repetitions or time) or static holds (weight x time) or equipment that measures and displays force during Isometric Hold.

When testing your Isometric Hold performance, it is essential to perform the exercises in the same manner each time, including the same repetition cadence, range of motion, and positioning, among other factors. Without this standardization, you won't be able to figure out whether changes in performance were due to improvements in functional ability or changes in the testing method itself.

Another way is to watch changes in goal-specific measurements, such as your weight, body composition, body part circumference measurements, clothing fit, and subjective evaluation of how you look and feel. This approach may be more practical for individuals who are unable to perform the exercises dynamically due to injuries or joint or neurological conditions.

A related disadvantage of Isometric Holds is that, without the visual feedback you get when performing exercises dynamically or using equipment that measures and displays your force input, you may be tempted to hold back instead of contracting as intensely as you should, particularly during the most challenging third phase. To overcome this, it is essential to look inward for motivation and stay focused on your goals. When your muscles are burning, your heart is pounding, and your lungs are on fire, and you are tempted to hold back, you must remember what you are working for and why it is more important to you than avoiding the temporary discomfort of intense exercise. Your results are directly proportional to the effort you put into each exercise, so giving it your best effort is essential to achieving the best possible results.

This book's full-body workout focuses on exercises that can be performed with a tow strap, rope or tie-down strap or even old dog leash bought inexpensively online or at any home improvement store. They are easily portable and can be carried in a gym bag, backpack, travel bag, or purse. While yielding isometric static holds can also effectively train all the major muscle groups using only bodyweight, they require a slightly more complex modulation of leverage and/or load distribution to accommodate all strength levels.

Isometric Holds automatically accommodate all strength levels, making it more time-efficient, particularly for people strong enough to perform bodyweight exercises unilaterally. (one hand or leg at a time).

45

For safety reasons, Bilateral Isometric Holds (working one side at a time) is preferable for individuals with neck and/or lower back problems, which may be worsened by performing unilateral exercises with the arms and/or legs, or those who struggle with unilateral lower body exercises due to balance or flexibility limitations. As a result, I encourage most of individuals who primarily train with bodyweight exercises to progress from bilateral squats to Isometric Hold squats rather than to unilateral squats.

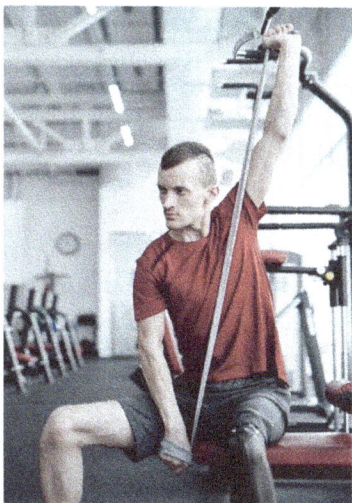

CARDIOVASCULAR AND METABOLIC CONDITIONING

Cardiovascular and metabolic conditioning can be effectively improved through strength training when performed with high intensity and sufficient duration. In fact, the improvements can be equal or greater than those achieved through traditional low-intensity endurance activities and sprint interval training.

The key factors in the metabolic cost and cardiovascular demands of an exercise are the amount of contracting muscle, the intensity of contraction, and the duration of the exercise, also known as force over time. It is not dependent on the specific type of movement, or the amount of visible movement produced. The heart is simply responding to the metabolic work being done and working harder to deliver oxygen and nutrients to the working muscles and remove waste products.

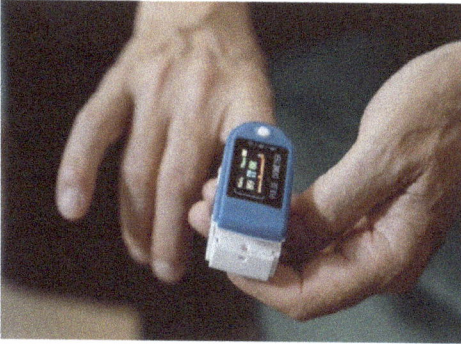

To achieve a significant elevation in heart rate and maintain it during a workout, it is recommended to include compound exercises that involve multiple joints and large muscle groups.

By performing these exercises with high intensity and transitioning quickly between them, one can achieve a substantial cardiovascular and metabolic effect. For example, performing six compound exercises can elevate heart rate to over 85% of predicted HRmax, while simple exercises for smaller muscle groups like neck flexors and extensors have only a minor effect, raising heart rate by only about 10% above resting levels. The greater muscle mass involved in compound exercises is the key to their enhanced cardiovascular and metabolic effects.

A compound exercise is a type of strength training exercise that involves multiple joints and muscle groups working together to perform a movement. This is in contrast to isolation exercises, which involve only one joint and a single muscle group. Compound exercises typically recruit more muscle fibers and require more energy and effort to perform than isolation exercises, making them an efficient and effective way to build overall strength and muscle mass.

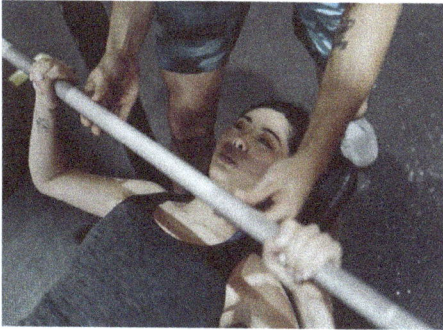

Examples of compound exercises include squats, deadlifts, bench press, pull-ups, and lunges.

Some added examples of compound exercises:

Shoulder press: This exercise works the shoulders, triceps, and upper back.

Barbell rows: This exercise targets the back, biceps, and core muscles.

Dips: This exercise primarily works the chest, triceps, and shoulders, but also engages the back and core muscles.

Pull-ups/chin-ups: These exercises work the back, biceps, and shoulders.

Lunges: This exercise primarily targets the legs, but also works the glutes, core, and lower back.

Deadlifts: This exercise works the entire posterior chain, including the hamstrings, glutes, lower back, and traps.

Bench press: This exercise primarily targets the chest, but also works the triceps, shoulders, and upper back.

Squats: This exercise primarily targets the legs, but also engages the glutes, core, and lower back.

The concept of strength transfer has been a common criticism of isometric training. Some argue that strength gains achieved through isometric exercises are specific to the positions trained and do not transfer to full-range strength. However, this assertion is not entirely correct.

Studies on the specificity of strength gains to the position trained have yielded mixed results. Some studies show that strength improvements are limited to only 15 to 20 degrees of the joint position trained. Other studies show full-range strength increases, and some studies, such as those conducted by MedX at the University of Florida in the 1990s, demonstrate that different people respond differently to isometric training. Most participants experienced position-specific strength increases, but a few improved strength over the full range of motion. To be safe, with my workouts I have concluded that an Isometric hold will cover 50% of your full range of motion. Most, if not all of the time when I do a hold now, **I use a**

two position Isometric hold. One in the Isometric position going right into a hold in the eccentric position. That gives me a full coverage.

However, based on years of experience training people with both isometric and dynamic exercises, it is suspected that a large part of the specificity in test results is due to some exercises having significant variation in the relative involvement of different muscles over the full range of motion. Additionally, a lack of skill in dynamic exercise performance among subjects who were only trained isometrically could be a factor.

For example, if a muscle is significantly involved in only one part of the range of motion of an exercise and if that exercise is performed isometrically in a position where that muscle has little or no involvement, the strength in the part of the range of motion where that muscle is involved will not increase proportionally. This assumes no other exercises are being performed that involve the muscle in question, which is usually the case in studies where subjects only perform and are tested on one or two exercises. If the whole body is being trained isometrically using exercises for all major muscle groups, these relative weak spots in the range of motion of dynamic exercises would be eliminated.

This issue is more pronounced with compound exercises than simple ones, as more muscles are involved, and the actions of many of the muscles that move the shoulders and hips are position dependent.

For example, when the shoulders are flexed (elbows in front of the body), the lats extend the shoulders, and when the shoulders are extended (elbows behind the body), the lats flex the shoulders. This means that the lats are significantly involved at the beginning of both a compound row and a parallel bar dip but have little or no involvement once the elbows pass the body. Depending on body position, the lats can extend, flex, depress, retract, adduct, or internally rotate the shoulders and assist in trunk flexion, lateral flexion, rotation, and extension.

Regardless of the joint position or portion of the range of motion trained, if a muscle is contracting with a high intensity of effort, all of the motor units in that muscle will be involved and stimulated to increase in strength and size. If the strength of that muscle increases, it will be able to produce more force at any length, from a full stretch to full contraction. Thus, if isometrics result in position-specific strength increases in some exercises because of significant variation in the contribution of the different muscles involved over the range of motion, the solution is simply to perform enough variety of exercise for all the major muscle groups to be worked effectively.

It is also important to consider that since the skill of performing an exercise is highly specific and has a strong influence on test performance, subjects who have only trained isometrically will be at a disadvantage in dynamic tests compared to subjects who have trained dynamically.

In the experience of those who use isometric holds and static holds in their workouts and with clients, there has been no indication that strength gains are limited to the position trained. For example, Ken Hutchins a few years ago, many of his clients performed isometric holds on equipment specially designed for the purpose.

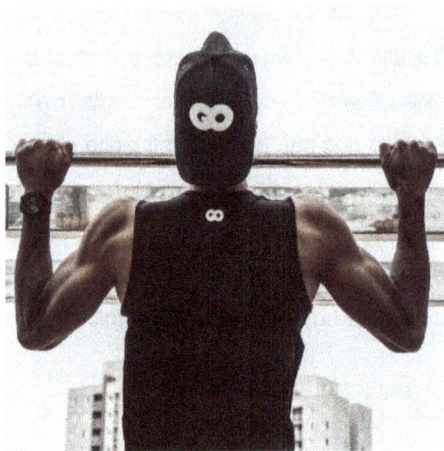

When it comes to safety considerations for Isometric Holds, it is important to note that if performed correctly, it is one of the safest forms of exercise. However, like any exercise method, improper technique can lead to injury. To minimize the risk of injury, it is crucial to follow certain guidelines.

As an Isometric hold practitioner and user, it is imperative to educate others about Isometric Holds and ensure they fully understand the proper technique before beginning. One important guideline is to gradually apply and increase force. During exercise, multiple muscle groups work together to achieve the desired movement. While stabilizing muscles are essential in maintaining proper positioning and balance, they can also produce more force than the target muscle group. This can cause injury if poor form is used.

For instance, during a standing barbell curl, the chest, shoulder, back, hip, and thigh muscles work to stabilize the upper arms, keep posture, and balance. If the back, hip, and thigh muscles contract with more force than needed, they can cause the back and hips to extend and transfer excessive force to the barbell, leading to bicep injury. Although the risk of injury during Isometric Hold arm curls is higher due to an immobile resistance, the same principles apply. Therefore, when performing Isometric Hold exercises, gradually apply force with the target muscles and avoid jerking or heaving at the weight.

Similarly, reactionary force produced by stabilizing muscles should increase gradually, rather than suddenly, to avoid overshooting the required amount of force and causing injury. It is also essential to increase force gradually between phases to minimize the risk of injury. By following these safety considerations, you can ensure a safe and effective workout with Isometric Hold.

Flexibility is a crucial factor in functional ability that cannot be significantly improved by isometric exercise. While strength training can enhance the range of motion for certain movements, isometric exercises should be performed near or past the mid-range position of the target muscles' range of motion, rather than in a stretched position. If you aim to improve or maintain your flexibility while only strength training isometrically, you will need to engage in supplementary stretching. This can be done after your workout or on non-workout days, and it may even enhance your strength gains.

Research conducted by Wayne Westcott found that those who performed high-intensity training with a 20-second static stretch after each exercise for the targeted muscles had a **20% greater increase in strength** over a ten-week period than those who did not stretch.

The purpose of stretching is not to lengthen your muscles or connective tissues, but rather to retrain your central nervous system to enable your muscles to lengthen further without resistance. The most effective way to do this is not to force your muscles into a deep stretch but to slowly and gradually move until you feel a stretch, then hold that position until your muscles relax. After your muscles have relaxed, repeat the process, gradually moving further until you feel a stretch again, and hold until your muscles relax. Stop when you reach a position where your muscles do not relax after holding for at least thirty seconds.

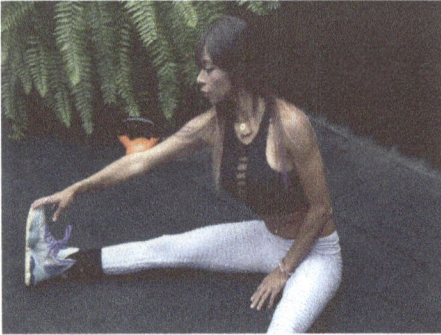

It is important to perform stretches in a position that does not require the stretched muscles to support your weight. For instance, stretching your hamstrings and calves while seated reduces the tension on those muscles.

When stretching, focus on feeling the stretch in your muscles, not your joints. If you experience a stretch in your joints, you may be doing the stretch incorrectly or

64

pushing yourself too hard. Lastly, stretching should never cause pain. If you experience any pain in your muscles or joints during stretching, stop immediately.

CAN ISOMETRIC HOLDS BE AS GOOD AS WEIGHTS?

Yes, isometric static holds can be an effective way to build strength, particularly in the muscles being targeted during the hold. Isometric exercises involve holding a position or contracting a muscle without any movement, which can be beneficial for building strength and improving muscular endurance.

During an isometric static hold, the muscle being targeted is contracted and held in a static position, which can help to improve muscle fiber recruitment and increase overall strength in that muscle. This type of exercise can also be helpful for developing stability and improving posture, as well as targeting specific muscles or muscle groups.

In fact, research has shown that isometric exercises can be as effective as traditional weightlifting for building strength and muscle mass. A study published in the **Journal of Strength and Conditioning Research found that isometric training was just as effective as dynamic training for improving strength in the quadriceps muscle group.**

Overall, isometric static holds can be a valuable addition to a strength training program, especially for individuals who want to avoid the joint stress that can come with traditional weightlifting. However, like any form of exercise, it's important to start with lighter resistance and gradually increase the intensity as you build strength and become comfortable with the exercise, and to use proper form and technique to reduce the risk of injury.

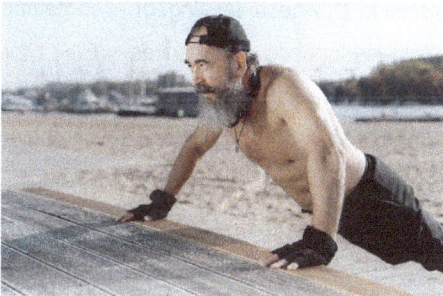

BREATHING

During exercise, it's common for individuals to hold their breath or perform a valsalva maneuver (forcefully exhaling while keeping the glottis closed). However, this habit can cause a rise in pressure in the thorax and abdomen, leading to a sudden and dangerous increase in blood pressure. Repeatedly doing this during exercise can result in dizziness, fainting, or even painful exercise-induced headaches (EIH) for some individuals. At best, holding your breath can lead to quicker fatigue during exercise.

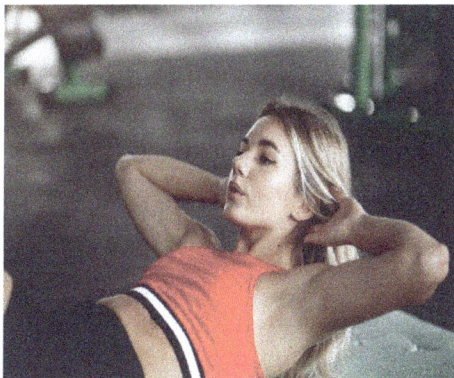

BREATHE ALWAYS BREATHE!

To prevent these negative effects, it's important to breathe continuously during exercise in a relaxed and natural manner. Breathe through a wide-open mouth without pursing your lips. Exhale with a "hah" sound instead of a "whoo" sound, and make sure the sound is solely the result of air moving through your mouth, without any contribution from your vocal cords. Avoid making any unnecessary noises like grunting or screaming, and remember that proper breathing should sound like panting, not like childbirth or torture.

Although some people may find it challenging to break the habit of holding their breath or performing a valsalva maneuver when contracting intensely, it's crucial to do so. If you realize that you're doing this, stop immediately and take a few deep breaths. If this happens frequently, try over-breathing by opening your mouth wide and breathing even faster. You may experience slight dizziness initially, but it's harmless and better than suffering from

EIH. Remember, the key to a successful workout is to keep breathing.

Isometric static holds are a form of resistance training that involves holding a specific position for a set period. Unlike dynamic movements, isometric holds do not involve any joint movement or range of motion. Instead, the muscle is contracted and held in a fixed position against an immovable object or a force that is equal to the maximum force that the muscle can produce. This creates tension in the muscle fibers, which can help to build strength, endurance, and stability.

Isometric holds can be used to target specific muscles or muscle groups, making them a useful addition to any strength training routine. For example, if you want to target your biceps, you can perform an isometric hold by holding a weight in front of your body with your elbows bent at a 90-degree angle. Similarly, if you want to target your core, you can hold a plank position for a set period of time.

One of the main benefits of isometric holds is that they can be done anywhere, without the need for any equipment. This makes them a convenient choice for people who do not have access to a gym or who are short of time. Additionally, isometric holds can be useful for people who are recovering from an injury or who have mobility issues, as they do not involve any joint movement.

To get the most benefit from isometric holds, it is important to gradually increase the duration and intensity of the holds over time. This can be done by increasing the amount of time that you hold the position, increasing the resistance or force that you are working against, or by incorporating multiple positions or angles into your routine. It is also important to remember that isometric holds should be incorporated alongside other forms of resistance training, such as dynamic movements and lifting weights, to promote overall muscle growth and strength.

Isometric holds involve holding a position where the targeted muscles are engaged and there's tension in the body without any movement. This means you are not lengthening or shortening your muscles nor moving up and down or side to side, just holding that position. The plank is an example of a quintessential static hold that can be challenging, even though you're not moving.

Certified experts recommend holding the position as long as you can keep proper form, as poor form can lead to injury. **Beginners can start with shorter holds of 5-7 seconds** and gradually work their way up to longer holds over time. For planks, a beginner can start with 10-15 seconds and gradually increase the hold time up to 1 minute. Many experts agree that Isometric holds over 20 seconds have no more success than 10-15 second holds. The muscle will fatigue fast, after 15 seconds.

The Introductory Isometric Hold workout is an effective full-body exercise routine that requires nothing but a strap and your own bodyweight, making it a convenient and accessible workout choice for anyone, anywhere. This workout is designed to safely and effectively train all the major muscle groups in the body, making it a well-rounded workout possibility.

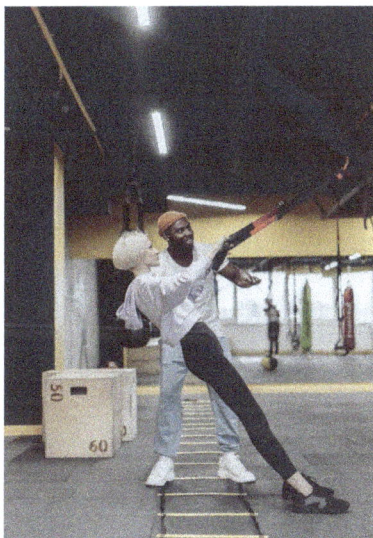

The workout consists of ten exercises that target various muscle groups, including the glutes, hamstrings, quadriceps, upper back, back of the shoulders, biceps, abs, chest, triceps, shoulders, upper traps, lower back, calves, front and back of the neck, and forearms. Each exercise involves holding a static position for a set period, which is known as an isometric hold. These holds are performed for a duration that is right for your fitness level, and they provide a challenging workout that helps to build strength and endurance.

BASIC ISOMETRIC HOLD WORKOUT

- The first exercise in the workout is the squat, which targets the glutes, hamstrings, and quadriceps.

- The stiff-legged deadlift, which targets the glutes, hamstrings, and lower back.

- This exercise is followed by the pulldown, which focuses on the upper back, back of the shoulders, biceps, and abdominal muscles.

- The compound row targets the upper back, back of the shoulders and traps, and biceps.

- The pullover is the seventh exercise in the workout, which targets the upper back, back of the shoulders, chest, and abs.

- The chest press is targeting the chest, front of the shoulders, and triceps.

- The shoulder press is the fifth exercise, which targets the shoulders, upper traps, and triceps.

- The triceps extension targets the triceps, and the chest press targets the chest, front of the shoulders, and triceps.

- The Arm curls, which target the biceps

- The Heel raise, which targets the calves.

- The final two exercises in the workout target the neck muscles and forearms respectively, with the neck flexion and extension exercise and grip and wrist flexion/extension exercise.

The Introductory Isometric Hold workout is a great choice for anyone looking for a challenging, yet convenient and accessible workout routine that targets all major muscle groups in the body. Whether you're a beginner or an experienced athlete, this workout can help you achieve your fitness goals and improve your overall health and well-being.

MACHINES

When it comes to performing Isometric Holds on machines, it's essential to use proper positioning for optimal safety and effectiveness. In general, it's recommended to use the same positions as you would for the corresponding Isometric Hold exercises performed with a strap. This typically means finding the midpoint of your range of motion where there is enough overlap of myofibrils for the targeted muscles to contract forcefully but not so much that you risk cramping.

It's important to note that when performing compound pushing movements like leg, chest, and shoulder presses, the leverage of the machine will prevent you from exerting too much pressure on your joints. This is especially important for those with a history of joint issues or injuries. For Isometric Hold leg presses and heel raises, it's crucial to use machines that allow you to load through your hips, like belt squats and heel raises. This will minimize the risk of injuring your lower back by preventing you from loading through your shoulders and spine.

For simple arm exercises like curls and triceps extensions, your elbows should be flexed at approximately ninety degrees. This will ensure that you are targeting the right muscles and prevent unnecessary strain on your joints. Similarly, for simple leg exercises like knee flexion and extension, your knees should be flexed at about forty-five degrees.

In summary, proper positioning is key to getting the most out of Isometric Hold exercises on machines. By finding the right range of motion and using machines that support safe loading, you can minimize the risk of injury and maximize the benefits of your workout.

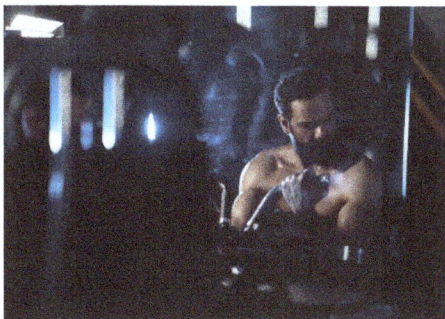

EQUIPMENT

In all my years of training I have come to love certain types of equipment that worked for me in my workouts. You have to remember when I started lifting the only equipment you had was a leather lifting belt. There were no water bottles, bench shirts, compression shorts or shirts. I have seen many products come through the gym, many of them just flat-out crap. In this chapter I will share with you some of the gear I came to love and use for the past forty years.

FAT GRIPZ

When I first heard about Fat Gripz, I thought they may have something there. A strong grip is crucial to not only working out, but it's also a sign of your overall fitness and strength. I ordered a pair. I put Fat Gripz right to work on my bar. I was amazed how they worked the forearm muscles while I was gripping. I found myself using them on my band handles and on my dumbbells as well as my bar. They became a regular part of my workouts. The real kick for me was when I found a unique way to use them all together. I went out to mow the lawn, jumped on the riding mower with the Fat Gripz wrapped around the steering wheel of the mower. My plan, to do some grip strength exercises while mowing. I didn't want to carry my expensive aluminum grippers, I thought these would be easy to store on the steering wheel. In the hour it takes mowing I knew I could get in a good five sets of grip squeezes. I didn't worry if they got wet or grass on them. The result was amazing! I had such a forearm pump from mowing with them on the steering wheel, I took them out every time I mowed!

Now, I use my Fat Gripz when I mow, I take them with me when I am driving as well. No better time to work forearms, than on an hour drive while stuck in the car. In fact, my

Fat Gripz are with me more than they are in the gym! I had to purchase another pair! I would say there is no better piece of gear than The Fat Gripz for building forearm and bicep size. I swear by them. In fact, I love them so much, I emailed the company to tell them I had to put them in this book. Matt was a major help. They gave me the green light to talk about this wonderful product!

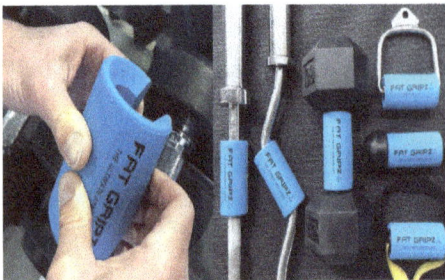

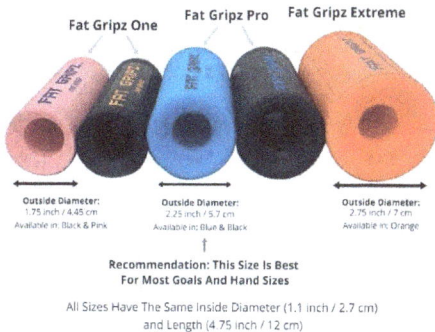

Fat Gripz One   Fat Gripz Pro   Fat Gripz Extreme

Outside Diameter:
1.75 inch / 4.45 cm
Available in: Black & Pink

Outside Diameter:
2.25 inch / 5.7 cm
Available in: Blue & Black

Outside Diameter:
2.75 inch / 7 cm
Available in: Orange

↑
Recommendation: This Size Is Best
For Most Goals And Hand Sizes

All Sizes Have The Same Inside Diameter (1.1 inch / 2.7 cm)
and Length (4.75 inch / 12 cm)

The theory behind fat gripz is that Fat Gripz Activates more muscle fibers meaning more muscle growth from every rep (no more wasted reps!) Increases grip strength, meaning you can use more weight on all exercises (no more weak links!)

I absolutely LOVE my Fat Gripz. Hey, don't take my word for it, visit their website and see who's using them.

The research has shown that using thick grip implements [Fat Grips] recruits more motor units [muscle fibers] especially in the elbow flexors [biceps and brachialis]. That means training with thicker diameter handles will build bigger, stronger arms."

CHARLES POLIQUIN

Trainer of over 400 Olympic athletes, Olympic medalists in 17 different sports and many bodybuilders and stars of the NFL and NHL

A big limiting factor in CrossFit is your grip strength affecting everything from Olympic lifts to pull-ups - do as much axle bar or FatGripz work as possible to fix this."

DMITRY KLOKOV

Olympic weightlifting champion and CrossFit expert.

fatgripz.com

To perform the exercises outlined in this book, you will need a sturdy, non-elastic strap that is approximately two inches in width and twice your height. The ideal width ensures that the strap will not dig into your body when pulled against any part, while still being comfortable to grip. The length should be long enough to execute exercises like the shoulder press and triceps extension while standing, without getting all tangled during other movements. If you prefer to perform the exercises while seated or kneeling, the strap can be shortened to one and a half times your height and placed under your hips instead of under your feet.

I use an auto tow strap or a nylon suspension strap. A rope or nylon dog leash will work. Minimum length of ten feet, should work unless you are tall. However, most auto towing and tie-down straps are strong enough to support Isometric Hold exercises, so you do not need to be concerned about the strength of the strap. After cutting the strap to your desired length, you can prevent fraying by wrapping the cut end with hockey tape. Another favorite I always have on hand is hockey tape. Not just any hockey tape. I ordered Howie's Hockey tape online. It comes in a

few assorted colors to match your color
scheme.

howieshockeytape.com

You can easily purchase the straps at home improvement or automotive parts stores, or online at an affordable price.

I purchased two sets of World Fit suspension straps. They are very rugged and have really nice, thick heavy-duty handles.

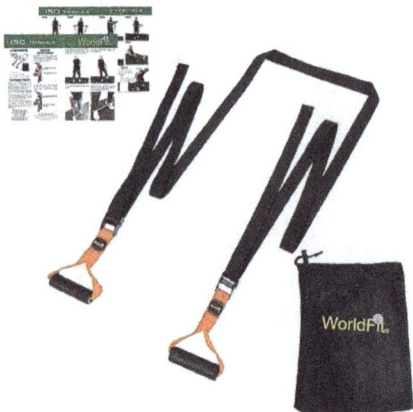

worldfit.com

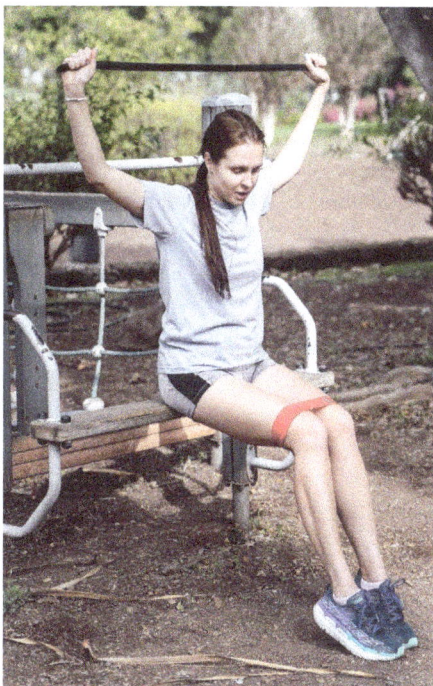

SIMPLE RULES

The following are some general guidelines for achieving best performance during your workouts:

Perform only one set of each exercise with high intensity of effort. This approach can stimulate improvements in strength and size of all the muscles worked and cardiovascular and metabolic conditioning. (Additional sets are often counterproductive and not necessary at the start)

Rest only long enough between exercises to avoid becoming out of breath, light-headed, or nauseated. There are some that say a 2-minute rest between sets is smart. To me that's far too long. Waiting that long will take all of the blood back out of the muscle. I use a 30 second rest.

Move slowly during exercises and quickly between them.

Allow your body enough time between workouts to recover from and produce the adaptations stimulated by exercise.

Overtraining can lead to plateau or even regression. Most people can perform two to three full-body workouts per week on non-consecutive days. Always remember that as we age, we lose muscle mass. The smart thing to do is to go to a 3-day workout to keep the muscles you have engaged.

If you are training with a high intensity of effort, more than this can quickly lead to overtraining. Some people's bodies recover and adapt more slowly, and they may require fewer exercises and more recovery days between workouts.

If you experience symptoms of overtraining, such as fatigue, depression, difficulty concentrating, frequent illness, or loss of motivation to train, reduce your workout volume or frequency.

You can reduce your workout volume by skipping a few workouts to allow your body enough time to recover, or by substituting fewer demanding exercises that target fewer and smaller muscle groups for one or two of the more demanding compound exercises.

To avoid completely removing any exercises from your program, you can alternate between some exercises and substitute for different exercises on alternating workouts.

If you're not getting noticeable results from your workouts, not making progress on occasional dynamic workouts, or experiencing symptoms of overtraining, don't be afraid to reduce your workout volume and/or frequency. Don't be afraid to change the order of your exercises if you find that you are not feeling the results. Or even adding in new exercises.

Remember that exercise stimulates your body to produce improvements as an adaptive response so that the next time your body encounters a similar stress, it is capable of handling it more easily. So, be patient and consistent with your workouts, and always listen to your body.

BUILDING MUSCLE

Isometric static holds are a form of resistance training that involves holding a specific position for a set period. Unlike dynamic movements, isometric holds do not involve any joint movement or range of motion. Instead, the muscle is contracted and held in a fixed position against an immovable object or a force that is equal to the maximum force that the muscle can produce. This creates tension in the muscle fibers, which can help to build strength, endurance, and stability.

Isometric holds can be used to target specific muscles or muscle groups, making them a useful addition to any strength training routine. For example, if you want to target your biceps, you can perform an isometric hold by holding a weight in front of your body with your elbows bent at a 90-degree angle. Similarly, if you want to target your core, you can hold a plank position for a set period of time.

One of the main benefits of isometric holds is that they can be done anywhere, without the need for any equipment. This makes them a convenient option for people who do not have access to a gym or who are short of time. Additionally, isometric holds can be useful for people who are recovering from an injury or who have mobility issues, as they do not involve any joint movement.

To get the most benefit from isometric holds, it is important to gradually increase the duration and intensity of the holds over time. This can be done by increasing the amount of time that you hold the position, increasing the resistance or force that you are working against, or by incorporating multiple positions or angles into your routine. It is also important to remember that isometric holds should be incorporated alongside other forms of resistance training, such as dynamic movements and lifting weights, to promote overall muscle growth and strength.

HEAT FACTOR

In order to avoid overheating during exercise, it is important to be aware of the negative effects that an increase in body temperature can have on your muscles and brain. Higher temperatures can cause fatigue and reduce focus and willpower, which can all impede your ability to work out at a high intensity. Furthermore, overheating can lead to various health risks such as heat cramps, fainting, heat exhaustion, and even heat stroke. While an increase in body temperature is inevitable during exercise, there are several measures you can take to minimize the risk.

One strategy is to exercise in a cool environment. If you are training indoors with air conditioning, this won't be an issue, but if you are training outdoors in a warm or hot climate, it is best to work out either early in the morning or late at night to avoid the hottest parts of the day. Whether you are training indoors or outdoors, if you have access to a power outlet, it is a great idea to use a fan to help prevent overheating. In fact, even in a cool environment, it is important to stay cool by dressing in light, breathable clothing that doesn't restrict your movement. Avoid wearing anything on your head that could interfere with heat dissipation unless it is necessary for religious reasons.

If you are unable to exercise in a cooler environment, there is a trick you can use to reduce body temperature. Holding a frozen water bottle between the palms of your hands between exercises has been shown to help extract heat from the palms and reduce body temperature, delaying fatigue and improving exercise performance.

Finally, it is crucial to stay well hydrated before and after your workout, regardless of your environment. Drinking plenty of fluids will help regulate your body temperature and prevent overheating. By following these guidelines, you can avoid overheating and safely exercise at a high intensity.

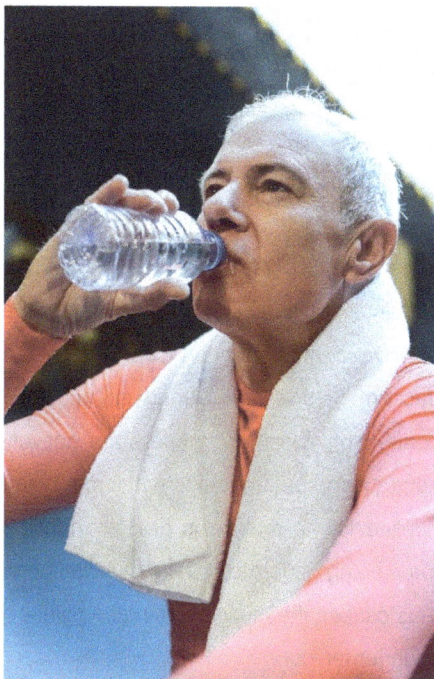

3 MUSCLE MOVEMENTS ANGLES
(ECCENTRIC, ISOMETRIC CONCENTRIC)

Eccentric: Eccentric contractions occur when a muscle is lengthening while still under tension. This usually happens when you are lowering weight, such as the downward phase of a bicep curl or the descent of a squat. During an eccentric contraction, the muscle fibers are actively contracting, but the external force being applied to the muscle is greater than the force being generated by the muscle fibers. This causes the muscle to lengthen while it is under tension.

Eccentric contractions are known to cause more muscle damage and soreness than other types of contractions. They can also generate greater force than concentric contractions, making them useful for improving strength and power.

Isometric: Isometric contractions occur when a muscle is generating force but there is no change in muscle length. This usually happens when you are holding a position or resisting an external force without moving. For example, holding a plank position or pushing against a wall. During an isometric contraction, the muscle fibers are actively contracting, but the external force being applied to the muscle is equal to the force being generated by the muscle fibers. This causes the muscle to maintain its length while it is under tension.

Isometric contractions are useful for improving muscular endurance and stability, as they can help strengthen the muscles in a static position. They are also beneficial for improving joint stability and preventing injury. However, isometric exercises typically do not generate as much muscle growth as eccentric or concentric exercises, as there is no active lengthening or shortening of the muscle fibers.

Concentric: Concentric contractions occur when a muscle is shortening while still under tension. This usually happens when you are lifting a weight, such as the upward phase of a bicep curl or the ascent of a squat. During a concentric contraction, the muscle fibers are actively contracting and generating force that is greater than the external force being applied to the muscle. This causes the muscle to shorten while it is under tension.

Concentric contractions are typically associated with muscle hypertrophy (growth) because they generate tension on the muscle fibers, which can lead to micro-tears and subsequent repair and growth. They are also useful for improving muscular endurance and power.

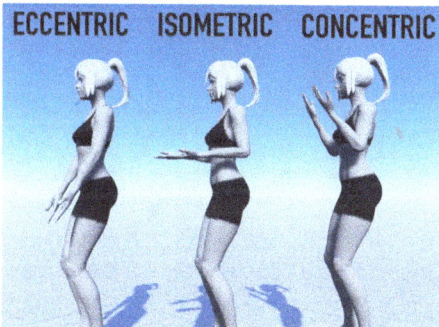

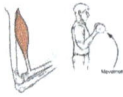

CONCENTRIC
(shortening)

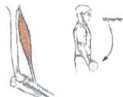

ECCENTRIC
(lengthening)

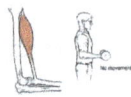

ISOMETRIC
(no movement)

EXERCISES

LEGS

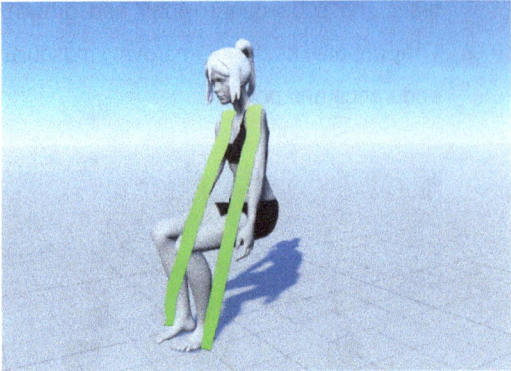

Squatting is a popular exercise that targets the lower body muscles such as glutes, hamstrings, and quadriceps. To perform a squat, start by standing with your feet shoulder-width apart. You can use a strap for added resistance and support. Place the strap around the back of your waist so that it sits just on top of your glutes, not higher on your lower back.

Cross the ends of the strap over each other in front of you. Hold the strap near the ends and begin to squat down slowly until your knees are bent at a 90-degree angle. Keep your back straight, chest lifted, and your weight centered over your heels.

Once you reach the bottom of your squat, loop the strap under your heels and pull it to remove the slack. This will create tension in the strap, which will help you maintain proper form and target your lower body muscles more effectively.

As you start to stand up, push through your heels, focusing on driving your hips up into the belt while contracting your glutes, hamstrings, and quadriceps. The strap will help you maintain proper form and keep your core engaged throughout the movement.

In addition to squatting, **isometric hold training can be a fantastic way to improve your overall strength and endurance.**

One exercise that is particularly effective for building upper body strength is the pulldown. This exercise can be performed with a bar at head height if available.

To perform the front pulldown, start by standing with your feet shoulder-width apart and your hands gripping the bar with an overhand grip. Keep your elbows close to your body and your shoulders down and back. Gently pull the bar down towards your chest, keeping your elbows close to your body and your shoulders down and back.

PULLDOWN

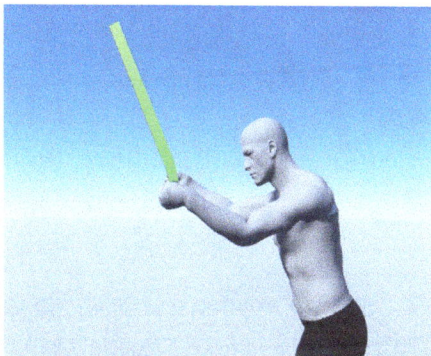

Once you reach your chest, hold the bar in place for a few seconds before slowly releasing it back to the starting position. Repeat for several reps, focusing on maintaining proper form and keeping your core engaged throughout the movement.

CALVES

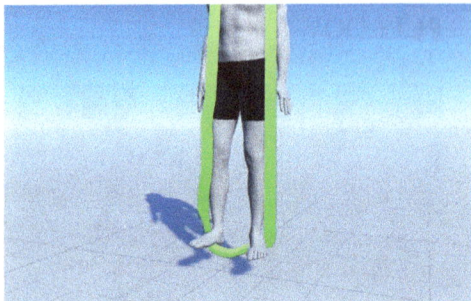

The heel raise exercise is a great way to build strength in your calf muscles, which are essential for many daily activities and sports. To perform this exercise, you will need a strap or resistance band.

To begin, stand with your feet shoulder-width apart and wrap the strap around the back of your waist, ensuring that it sits just on top of your glutes and not higher on your lower back. Cross the ends of the strap over each other in front of you.

Next, hold the strap near the ends and bend your knees slightly. Loop the strap under the balls of your feet and pull it to remove any slack. This will ensure that the resistance is evenly distributed across both feet.

Once you are in position, slowly raise your heels off the ground by pushing through the balls of your feet. Focus on contracting your calf muscles as you lift and hold the contraction at the top of the movement for a few seconds.

Lower your heels back down to the ground and repeat for a set number of repetitions. It's important to maintain good form throughout the exercise, keeping your core engaged and your back straight.

To make this exercise more challenging, you can increase the resistance of the strap or hold a weight in each hand. Alternatively, you can perform the exercise on one leg at a time to really target each calf individually.

Incorporating heel raises into your regular workout routine can help to improve your calf strength and overall lower body power, making it easier to perform activities like running, jumping, and squatting.

STRAP DEADLIFT

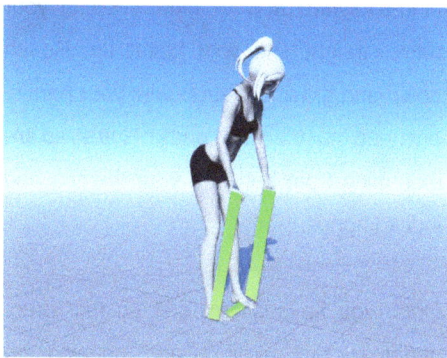

The Stiff-Legged Deadlift is a popular exercise that primarily targets the posterior chain muscles, including the hamstrings, glutes, and lower back. This exercise is performed by standing with your feet approximately shoulder-width apart and looping a strap under the middle of your feet.

To begin, bend your knees slightly and hinge forward at your hips, keeping your back straight and your chest up. Reach down and grasp the strap with your hands, ensuring that the loose ends of the strap are extending from between your thumbs and index fingers.

Once you have a firm grip on the strap, begin to pull straight up, focusing on contracting your hamstrings, glutes, and lower back. As you lift the strap, keep your back straight and your core engaged to avoid rounding or arching your back.

At the top of the movement, pause for a moment to squeeze your glutes and ensure that you are fully engaging your posterior chain muscles. Slowly lower the strap back down to knee height, maintaining control and proper form throughout the movement.

To maximize the benefits of the Stiff-Legged Deadlift, it is important to use proper form and technique. Keep your back straight and your core engaged throughout the exercise, and focus on using your hamstrings, glutes, and lower back to lift the weight. As you become more comfortable with the exercise, you can gradually increase your weight to continue challenging your muscles and promoting growth and development.

Incorporating the Stiff-Legged Deadlift into your workout routine can help to improve your overall strength, stability, and balance. By targeting your posterior chain muscles, this exercise can help to improve your posture, reduce your risk of injury, and enhance your athletic performance.

BACK ROW

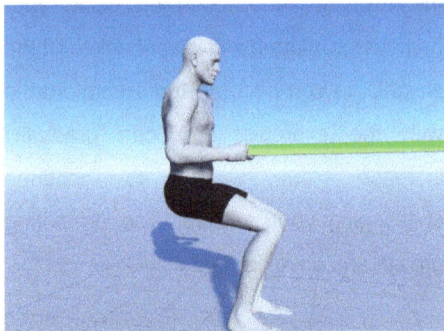

The Compound Row is an effective exercise that targets multiple muscle groups in your upper body. This exercise is great for building strength, improving posture, and enhancing overall fitness.

To perform the Compound Row, sit with your legs straight in front of you and your back straight. Loop a resistance band or strap under the middle of your feet and hold the loose ends of the strap with your thumbs and index fingers. Your arms should be angled slightly away from your sides, and your elbows should be bent at approximately ninety degrees.

Before beginning the exercise, engage your core muscles and take a deep breath. As you exhale, pull the strap towards your chest while contracting the muscles in your upper back, shoulders, and biceps. Focus on pulling your shoulder blades down and back, keeping your elbows close to your sides, and squeezing your shoulder blades together at the top of the movement. Hold the tension for a few seconds and then slowly release the strap, returning to the starting position. Repeat for several repetitions, focusing on maintaining proper form and breathing throughout the exercise.

To increase the intensity of the Compound Row, you can adjust the resistance of the strap or use a heavier weight. You can also vary the grip by using an overhand or underhand grip, or by gripping the strap with your palms facing each other.

Incorporating the Compound Row into your regular workout routine can help you build strength in your upper body, improve your posture, and enhance your overall fitness level. As with any exercise, it's important to start with a warm-up and to consult with a fitness professional if you have any concerns or underlying medical conditions.

PULLOVER

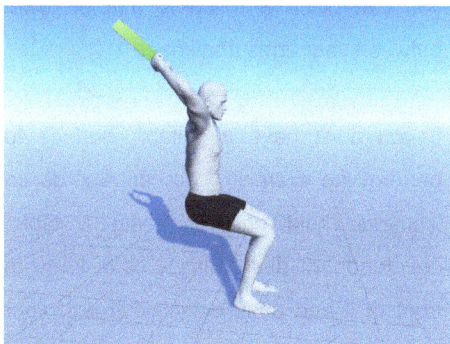

The exercise known as the pullover can be performed in a squatting or sitting position with your knees bent. Start by placing the backs of your elbows on top of your knees and slightly flex your trunk so that your shoulders are at about a 90-degree angle. Now push down on your knees with the backs of your arms, while focusing on contracting the muscles in your upper back, shoulders, and abs. To reduce discomfort, you can place a rolled-up mat or towel between your arms and knees.

If you don't have a suitable surface to perform the exercise, you can also do an isometric hold pullover using a table, countertop, or desk. Simply sit or kneel in front of it and push down on it with your elbows, engaging the same muscle groups as in the traditional pullover. It's worth noting that the pullover exercise can be beneficial for strengthening the upper body and improving posture. However, as with any exercise, it's important to use proper form and start with lighter weights or less resistance before gradually increasing intensity.

PULLDOWN

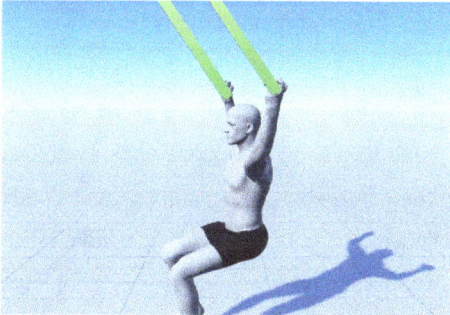

A pulldown is an effective exercise that targets the muscles in your upper back, shoulders, and biceps. It can be performed using a bar at head height or by looping a strap over a higher structure, such as a tree branch or a strong bar. If you're indoors, you can tie an overhand knot in the center of the strap and anchor it over the top of a door on the side it opens towards, ensuring that it's securely held against the top of the door frame when the door is closed.

To perform a pulldown, grip the strap at head height with the loose ends extending from between your thumbs and index fingers and your palms facing towards you. Keep your core engaged, your shoulders down and back, and your chest lifted. Then, pull down on the strap, focusing on contracting the muscles in your upper back, back of your shoulders, and biceps. Pause briefly at the bottom of the movement, then slowly release the tension as you raise the strap back up to the starting position.

To get the most out of your pulldowns, be sure to maintain proper form throughout the exercise. Keep your elbows close to your body, avoid arching your back or rounding your shoulders, and maintain a steady, controlled movement. As you become stronger, you can increase the resistance by using a heavier strap or by adding additional weight. With consistent practice, the pulldown can help you develop strong, toned upper body muscles and improve your overall fitness and health.

CHEST

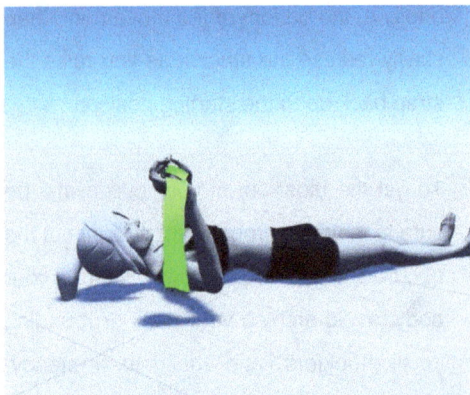

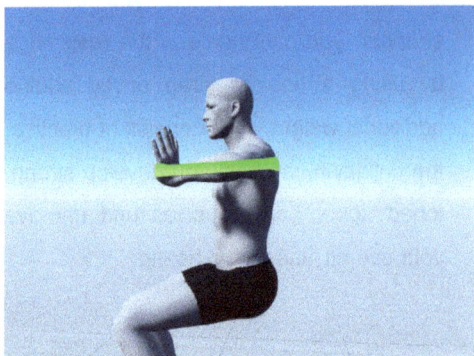

The chest press is a popular exercise that targets the muscles in the chest, shoulders, and triceps. It involves using a strap looped around the back and arms to create resistance as you push forward. This exercise is commonly performed with a resistance band or a cable machine but can also be done with a simple strap.

To perform the chest press, begin by looping the strap around your back, just below your shoulder blades. Next, grip the strap with both hands so that it is wrapped around the outside of your arms. The loose ends of the strap should extend from between your thumbs and index fingers.

With your arms angled slightly forward and away from your sides, bend your elbows to about ninety degrees. This is your starting position. From here, push straight forward, focusing on contracting the muscles in your chest, the front of your shoulders, and your triceps.

As you push forward, be sure to maintain proper form. Keep your shoulders down and back and engage your core muscles to stabilize your body. Exhale as you push, and inhale as you return to the starting position.

To maximize the effectiveness of the chest press, vary the angle of your arms and the amount of resistance used. You can also perform this exercise with one arm at a time, or with a staggered stance for added balance and stability.

Incorporating the chest press into your workout routine can help to strengthen and tone your upper body, improve your posture, and enhance your overall fitness level. As with any exercise, be sure to warm up properly beforehand, and consult with a fitness professional if you have any questions or concerns about your form or technique.

SHOULDERS

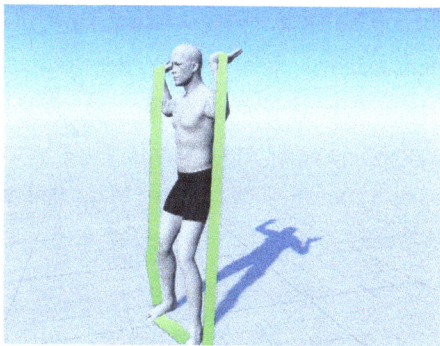

The shoulder press is a resistance exercise that targets the muscles of the shoulders, upper traps, and triceps. It is typically performed using a resistance band or strap, although it can also be done with dumbbells or a barbell.

To perform the shoulder press with a resistance band or strap, start by standing with your feet approximately shoulder-width apart. Loop the strap under the middle of your feet and grip it so that it is wrapped around the back of your arms with the loose ends extending from the pinky edge of your hands. Your arms should be angled forward slightly and parallel to the ground, with your elbows bent slightly more than ninety degrees.

Next, push straight up, focusing on contracting your shoulders, upper traps, and triceps. Be sure to keep your core engaged and your back straight throughout the movement. Exhale as you push up, and inhale as you lower back down.

If your resistance band or strap is not long enough to perform the exercise while standing, you can also do it while sitting or kneeling with the strap looped under your hips. In this variation, keep your back straight and your core engaged, and focus on maintaining proper form throughout the movement.

The shoulder press is a great exercise for building strength and muscle mass in the shoulders and upper body. It can be done as part of a full-body workout or as a standalone exercise for the upper body. As with any resistance exercise, be sure to start with a weight or resistance level that is right for your fitness level, and gradually increase the intensity and duration of the exercise as you get stronger.

LATERAL RAISE

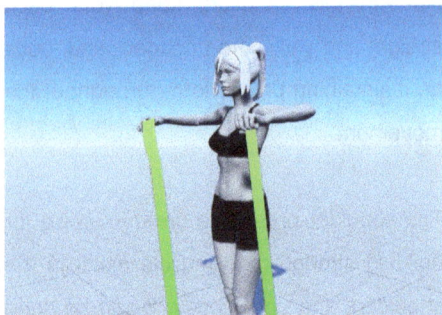

The lateral raise is a popular exercise that targets the shoulder and upper back muscles, particularly the deltoids and trapezius. Here is a detailed guide on how to perform the lateral raise:

Start by standing with your feet shoulder-width apart and your core engaged.

Place a resistance band or strap under the middle of your feet and grip the ends of the strap with your thumbs and index fingers.

Keep your arms straight with a slight bend at the elbows and your palms facing your body.

Begin by raising your arms out to the sides and up, keeping them in line with your shoulders.

As you lift your arms, focus on contracting the muscles in your shoulders and upper back.

Pause at the top of the movement and hold for a second, then slowly lower your arms back down to the starting position.

Repeat for several repetitions, aiming for 2-3 sets of 10-15 reps.

Some tips to keep in mind while performing the lateral raise include:

Keep your neck and spine in a neutral position throughout the exercise.
Avoid arching your back or shrugging your shoulders.

Use a slow and controlled motion, rather than swinging your arms.

Exhale as you lift your arms and inhale as you lower them.

Incorporating the lateral raise into your workout routine can help improve shoulder and upper back strength and stability, which can be beneficial for everyday activities and other exercises.

TRICEPS

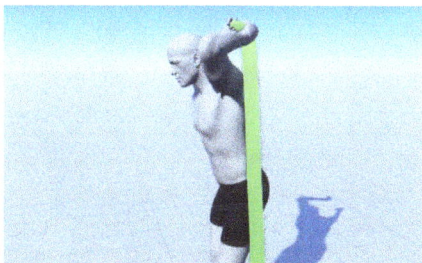

Triceps Extension is a popular exercise that targets the triceps, which are the muscles on the back of the upper arms. The exercise is usually performed with a resistance band or strap, making it a great option for people who prefer to workout at home or have limited access to equipment.

To perform a triceps extension, start by standing with your feet approximately shoulder-width apart. Loop the strap under the middle of your feet and grip the strap above and behind your head with the loose ends extending from the pinky edge of your hands. Your forearms should be parallel to the ground, and your elbows should be bent about ninety degrees.

From this starting position, push straight up, focusing on contracting your triceps. As you extend your arms, try to keep your elbows close to your head and avoid letting them flare out to the sides. Squeeze your triceps at the top of the movement, then slowly lower the strap back down to the starting position.

If you don't have a long enough strap to perform the exercise while standing, you can also do it while sitting or kneeling with the strap looped under your hips. Alternatively, if you have access to something overhead like a chin-up bar or door frame, you can secure the strap and perform the exercise while gripping it in front of you in the mid-range position of a cable triceps press down.

To make the exercise more challenging, you can increase the resistance by using a thicker or shorter strap, or by using dumbbells or a barbell instead. You can also vary the tempo of the exercise by performing it slowly and controlled or by adding explosive movements to challenge your muscles in different ways.

Incorporating triceps extensions into your workout routine can help you build stronger, more defined arms and improve your overall upper body strength and endurance. As with any exercise, it's important to use proper form, start with a light resistance and gradually increase the intensity as your muscles adapt, and to listen to your body and avoid pushing through pain or discomfort.

BICEP

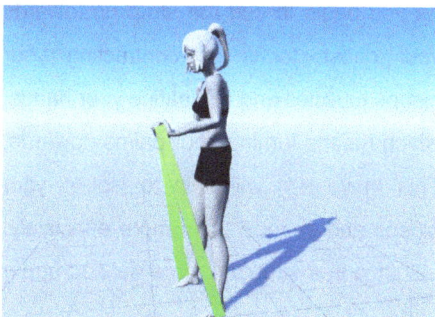

The arm curl is a simple yet effective exercise that targets the biceps muscles in your upper arms. To perform this exercise, you should stand with your feet shoulder-width apart and loop a strap under the middle of your feet. Next, you need to grip the strap with the loose ends extending between your thumbs and index fingers, while keeping your elbows close to your sides and bent at a ninety-degree angle.

As you begin to curl the strap up towards your chest, focus on contracting your biceps muscles and supinating your hands, which means turning your palms upwards. This movement will help to isolate your biceps and engage them more effectively, resulting in a stronger, more defined upper arm.

It's important to keep your movements slow and controlled throughout the exercise, avoiding any jerky or sudden motions that could put unnecessary strain on your muscles or joints. Start with a lighter weight or resistance band and gradually increase as you become more comfortable with the movement.

Incorporating arm curls into your regular workout routine can help to improve your upper body strength and tone your arms, making it a great exercise to include in your fitness regimen.

NECK

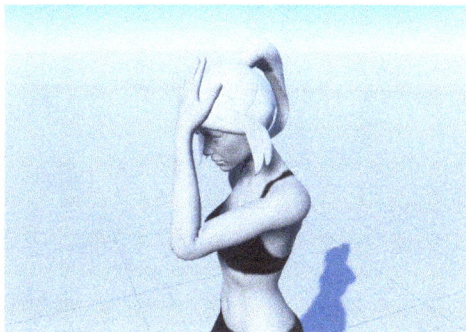

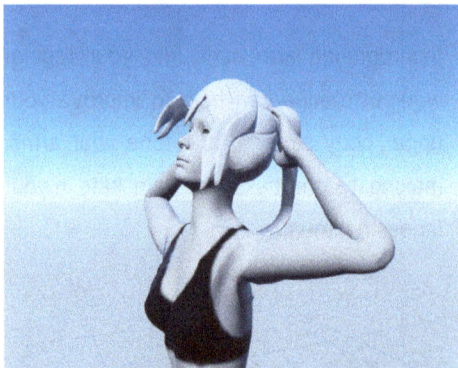

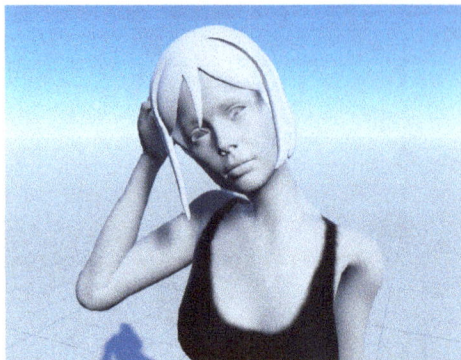

Neck flexion and extension are two essential exercises that help improve the strength and flexibility of the neck muscles. These exercises are particularly beneficial for individuals who sit for extended periods or those who suffer from neck pain and stiffness.

To perform neck flexion, start by holding your head in a neutral position, with your chin parallel to the ground. Next, place the heels of your palms on your forehead just above your eyebrows, ensuring that you do not place them below the eyebrows where the skin

is thinner and more delicate. Gently press your forehead forward and downwards into your palms while contracting the muscles in the front of your neck. Hold this position for a few seconds before releasing and repeating the exercise.

On the other hand, neck extension involves holding your head in a neutral position and wrapping a strap around the center of the back of your head. Ensure that the strap is level with your eyes and hold the ends of the strap in front of your head. Gently press your head back against the strap while contracting the muscles in the back of your neck, from the base of your skull down to between your shoulder blades. Hold this position for a few seconds before releasing and repeating the exercise.

It's worth noting that these exercises should be done in a controlled and gentle manner. Overdoing them may lead to muscle strain and soreness. Start with a few repetitions and gradually increase as you become more comfortable with the movements.

Additionally, it's advisable to consult with a healthcare professional before starting any new exercise routine, particularly if you have a history of neck injuries or chronic neck pain.

GRIP/ FOREARM

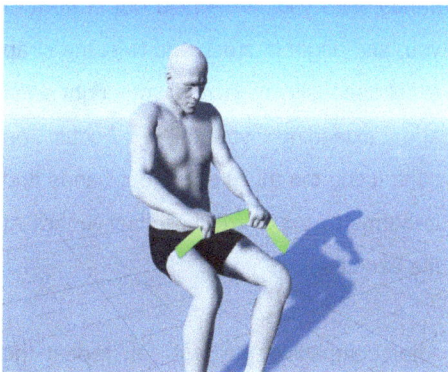

To effectively work on your grip and wrist flexion/extension, begin by taking a strap and folding it until it is slightly longer than the width of your shoulders. Then, grip the folded strap at shoulder width and twist the right side with an overhand motion while flexing your wrist until it reaches its limit.

Next, secure the folded strap with both hands, with your arms held out in front of you, and begin to crush and twist the strap simultaneously by flexing your right wrist and extending your left. Focus on contracting the muscles in your hands and forearms to maximize the effectiveness of the exercise.

After completing the first set, repeat the steps by twisting the strap in the opposite direction, flexing your left wrist and extending your right. This will ensure that both sides of your body receive equal attention and exercise.

Additionally, you can also perform hand supination and pronation exercises by using the strap. Extend your arms in front of you with your palms facing each other and shoulder-width apart. Hold the strap between your thumbs and forefingers to isometrically supinate both hands and hold it between your little fingers to isometrically pronate them.

It is important to note that grip and forearm exercises should always be performed at the end of your workout to avoid compromising your ability to grip during other exercises. By incorporating these exercises into your fitness routine, you can

develop stronger and more resilient grip
and wrist muscles.

AB/PLANK

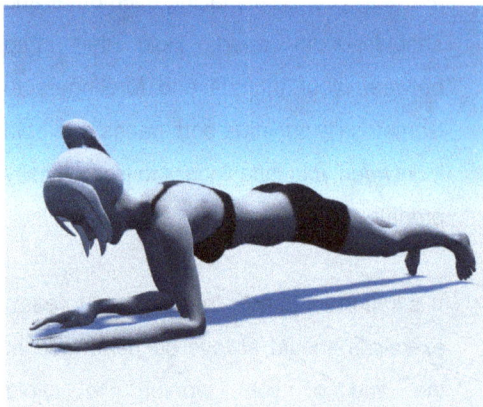

An isometric abdominal hold, also known as
the plank, is a great exercise for

strengthening your core muscles. Here's
how to perform it:

Start by getting into a push-up position with
your hands shoulder-width apart and your
arms straight.

Your body should be in a straight line from
your head to your heels, with your feet hip-
width apart.

Tighten your abdominal muscles and hold
this position for a specific amount of time,
starting with 10-20 seconds and gradually
increasing the duration as you get stronger.

Make sure to keep your hips in line with
your shoulders and your neck in a neutral
position.

Breathe deeply and evenly throughout the exercise.

To release the hold, slowly lower your body to the ground.

It's important to maintain proper form throughout the exercise to avoid injury and get the most out of the workout.

TRAINING FREQUENCY

The frequency and volume of your workouts play a crucial role in your body's ability to adapt and improve. Exercise itself does not directly lead to improvements, but rather stimulates your body to respond adaptively to the stress, resulting in improved strength, size, and other functional abilities. However, your body needs time to recover and produce these adaptations between workouts, and not allowing enough time for recovery can lead to overtraining and a plateau in progress or even regression.

To perfect workout frequency and volume, most people find that two to three full-body workouts per week on non-consecutive days' work best. However, the ideal frequency and volume can vary based on individual factors such as recovery rate, intensity of effort, and the need for rest days between workouts. Some individuals may require fewer exercises and more recovery time to avoid overtraining, while others may be able to handle more frequent or intense workouts.

It's important to check your workout performance over time and adjust your frequency and volume accordingly. If you experience unusually slow or no progress, it may be a sign that you need to adjust your workout frequency or volume. Other signs of overtraining include fatigue, depression, difficulty concentrating, frequent sickness, and loss of motivation. If you experience any of these symptoms, it may be time to reduce the volume or frequency of your workouts to allow your body to recover adequately. The easy thing to do is keep a small log and go back to it as a reference.

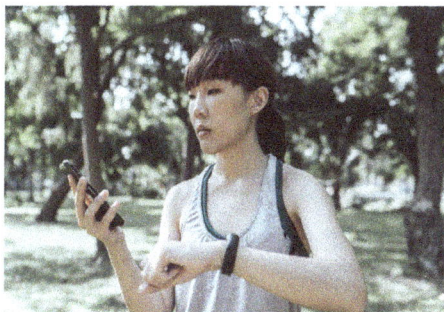

DO ISOMETRIC HOLDS WORK FOR SPEED SPORTS?

Explosiveness is an important aspect of athletic performance, especially in sports that require rapid acceleration or quick movements. Many athletes use isometric holds as part of their training to improve their explosive power. But can isometric holds really help build power?

The answer is yes. Isometric holds can increase muscular strength, which is directly related to power. Strength is the measure of the force your muscles can produce, while power is the measure of work performed over time. When your muscles are stronger, they can produce more force when contracting and accelerate your body or other objects you are pushing or pulling more rapidly.

This means you can perform the same amount of work in less time, or more work in the same amount of time, resulting in increased power. For example, if you can only press a weight of 100 pounds, you will not be able to press it quickly or many times per minute. However, if you double your strength to 200 pounds, you will be able to lift the same 100-pound weight more quickly and more times per minute.

It doesn't matter how you increase your strength, whether it's with fast or slow repetitions or through isometric holds. If you become stronger, you will become more powerful. This can have a significant impact on your athletic performance and help you to achieve your goals. By incorporating isometric holds into your training routine, you can build your strength and increase your power, ultimately improving your overall athletic performance.

ISOMETRIC HOLDS AND CALORIE BURNING

Isometric holds involve holding a specific position or posture for a period without moving. Examples of isometric exercises include planks, wall sits, and static lunges. These exercises are great for building strength and improving muscle endurance because they require you to engage your muscles and hold them in a contracted position.

However, isometric exercises don't typically burn as many calories as exercises that involve movement or aerobic activity. This is because calorie burning is directly related to the amount of movement and energy expended during an activity. Isometric holds, by their nature, involve minimal movement and energy expenditure, so they may not burn as many calories as other forms of exercise. With that said, doing longer holds 15 seconds plus with proper breathing will definitely take the wind out of your sails!

Isometric exercises can still be a valuable part of a fitness routine. By building strength and endurance through isometric holds, you may be better able to perform other exercises that do burn calories, such as cardio workouts or weight training. For example, if you can hold a plank for a longer period, you may be able to perform more reps of a weightlifting exercise, which can lead to greater calorie burning and muscle development.

Additionally, isometric exercises can be a good option for people who are recovering from an injury or who have joint pain. Since isometric exercises don't involve as much movement or impact on the joints, they can be a safer and more comfortable choice for some people.

In conclusion, while isometric exercises may not be the most effective method for burning calories, they can still be a useful addition to a fitness routine. By building strength and endurance through isometric holds, you may be able to perform other exercises that do burn calories, and they can also be a safer option for some people with joint issues.

ISOMETRICS FOR INJURY REHABBING

Isometric exercises can be particularly beneficial for rehabbing an injury because they can help to maintain muscle strength and range of motion without putting undue stress on the injured area. When a muscle is contracted isometrically, it generates tension without actually changing length, which can be useful in situations where movement is restricted or painful.

Here are some reasons why isometric exercises are commonly used for rehabbing injuries:

Builds strength: Isometric exercises can help to build and maintain muscle strength without putting undue stress on the injured area. By holding a position for a period, the muscle is forced to generate tension, which can help to maintain muscle mass and prevent atrophy.

Reduces pain: Isometric exercises can be a good option for individuals who are experiencing pain during movement, as they can help to reduce pain by minimizing movement around the injured area. By stabilizing the affected joint or muscle, isometric exercises can help to relieve pain and discomfort.

Improves range of motion: Isometric exercises can also be useful in improving range of motion by allowing the muscle to stretch without actually moving the joint. By holding a position for a period, the muscle is forced to lengthen, which can help to improve flexibility and mobility.

Low impact: Isometric exercises are low-impact and can be performed without the need for equipment, making them an accessible option for many individuals. They can also be modified to accommodate various levels of fitness and injury severity.

Overall, isometric exercises can be an effective tool for rehabbing an injury by maintaining muscle strength and range of motion, reducing pain, and improving overall function. However, it's important to work with a healthcare professional or physical therapist to develop a suitable exercise program that considers the specific needs and limitations of the individual.

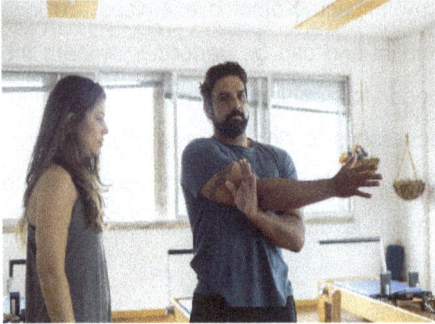

Isometric exercises, which involve contracting the muscles without joint movement, are indeed commonly used in rehabilitation for injuries and surgeries. Doctors and physical therapists often incorporate isometric exercises into treatment plans for several reasons:

Early-stage rehabilitation: Isometric exercises are often introduced in the initial stages of rehabilitation when active movement may be restricted or contraindicated. They allow patients to start engaging their muscles without putting excessive stress on healing tissues. This helps maintain muscle strength, prevent muscle atrophy, and stimulate blood flow to the injured area.

Muscle activation and recruitment: Isometric exercises target specific muscles or muscle groups, activating and recruiting them without placing excessive strain on the joints. By selectively activating the muscles around an injured area, doctors can help stabilize joints, improve muscle control, and restore normal movement patterns.

Pain management: Isometric exercises can be used as part of a pain management strategy. When muscles are contracted isometrically, they often produce an analgesic (pain-relieving) effect due to the release of endorphins. This can help alleviate pain and discomfort during the rehabilitation process.

Joint protection: Following an injury or surgery, it's important to protect the affected joint. Isometric exercises allow patients to strengthen the muscles around the joint without placing direct stress on the joint itself. This promotes joint stability and can help prevent further damage while supporting the healing process.

Gradual progression: Isometric exercises provide a controlled and graded approach to rehabilitation. As patients progress in their recovery, the intensity and duration of isometric contractions can be adjusted to accommodate their improving strength and function. This gradual progression helps ensure a safe and effective rehabilitation process.

Convenience and versatility: Isometric exercises can be performed in various positions and require little to no equipment, making them convenient for patients to perform both in clinical settings and at home. They can be tailored to target specific muscles or joint angles, allowing for a personalized rehabilitation program.

THE SAFETY FACTOR

Isometric holds can offer several safety benefits over free weights, particularly when it comes to joint stress and injury risk. Here are some of the ways in which isometric holds may be safer than free weights:

Reduced Joint Stress: Isometric holds involve static contractions of muscles without any joint movement. This can reduce the stress on joints, especially for individuals who may have pre-existing joint problems or injuries. In contrast, free weight exercises require movement through a range of motion, which can increase joint stress and risk of injury.

Controlled Range of Motion: Isometric holds allow you to control the range of motion and the amount of tension on your muscles. This can be especially helpful for individuals who are new to strength training or who have limited mobility. With free weights, it's possible to move through a range of motion that is beyond your current capabilities, increasing the risk of injury.

Reduced Risk of Accidents: Isometric holds can be done without any equipment or with minimal equipment, such as a wall or chair. This means that there is less risk of accidents or injuries caused by dropping heavy weights or mishandling equipment. In contrast, free weights require proper form and technique to prevent accidents or injuries.

Better Muscle Activation: Isometric holds can help activate deep stabilizing muscles that may not be targeted with free weights. This can help improve overall joint stability and reduce the risk of injuries caused by imbalances or weaknesses in these muscles.

Overall, isometric holds can offer a safe and effective alternative to free weights for individuals who may have joint problems, limited mobility, or who are new to strength training. However, it's important to note that both types of exercises have their benefits and limitations, and it's important to choose the type of exercise that best fits your goals and abilities.

THE COST FACTOR

Isometric holds can be a great way to strengthen and tone your muscles, and they can be done at home or at the gym. When considering the cost benefits of doing isometric holds at home versus going to the gym, there are a few factors to consider:

Equipment: Isometric holds can be done with little to no equipment, making them a cost-effective option for home workouts. However, if you prefer to use equipment such as a resistance band, chains or suspension straps, you may need to purchase these items for home use. On the other hand, a gym membership will typically provide access to a wide range of equipment without any additional costs.

Time: Going to the gym can take time out of your day, especially if you have to travel to and from the gym. Doing isometric holds at home can save you time and make it easier to fit exercise into your daily routine.

Motivation: Some people find that they are more motivated to exercise when they go to the gym and are surrounded by other people who are working out. Others may prefer the privacy and convenience of doing isometric holds at home.

Cost: The cost of a gym membership can vary widely depending on the location and type of gym. In general, doing isometric holds at home will be the most cost-effective option, as you won't have to pay for a gym membership or any equipment. However, if you already have a gym membership and enjoy going to the gym for other types of workouts, adding isometric holds to your routine may not add any other costs.

Overall, the cost benefits of doing isometric holds at home versus going to the gym will depend on your individual circumstances and preferences. Consider the factors listed above to figure out which way is best for you.

ISOMETRIC HOLD VERSUS DOING NOTHING

If there is one thing, I hope you take away from this book is that working out and exercising is not recreation, it's a way to keep your body and mind healthy! A healthy body and mind will extend your life. My books are not about making you look like a bodybuilder. They have so many customized drugs today, steroids are an art form on their own. The average person could never get that large. I know people tell me all the time they are worried that they will get too big and need a new wardrobe! Not going to happen with my programs. You will tone your muscles, look good and get strong.

The alternative to that is doing nothing, gaining 50 pounds, developing diabetes, high blood pressure and always feeling tired. Doing nothing will make you sick and frail as you get older! Let's look at the Isometric hold as a quick workout alternative.

Isometric holds, also known as isometric exercises, involve holding a position without any joint movement or muscle contraction. These exercises have been found to offer numerous benefits over doing no exercise at all. Here are some of the benefits of isometric holds:

Increased strength: Isometric holds can help increase your muscular strength, as your muscles are forced to contract without any movement. Over time, this can lead to improved strength and muscle tone.

Improved stability: Isometric holds can improve your body's stability and balance, as these exercises require you to maintain a stable position without any movement.

Increased endurance: Isometric holds can help increase your muscular endurance, as you must hold a position for an extended period of time. This can improve your ability to perform everyday activities and other physical activities.

173

Reduced risk of injury: Isometric holds can help reduce your risk of injury, as they can help strengthen the muscles around your joints, improving their stability and reducing the risk of joint-related injuries.

Improved mental focus: Isometric holds require a significant amount of mental focus, as you must keep a position for an extended period. This can help improve your mental focus and concentration.

Overall, while isometric holds may not provide the same benefits as dynamic exercises, they can still be a valuable addition to your exercise routine and provide numerous benefits over doing no exercise at all.

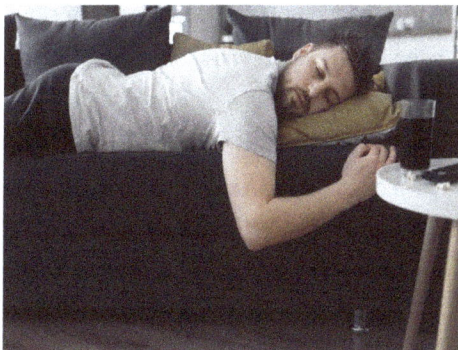

THE LIMP PROGRAM
Light Isometric Movement
Program

THE 911 HYSO 'DAYO'

As a side note to all the options. I developed
the 911 HYSO workout as opposed to doing
nothing at all. For the past two consecutive

175

spring seasons I developed massive sinus infections which turned into Acute Bronchitis. Taking a series of antibiotics while authoring this book, I also then developed a bacterial infection. I was looking at a good month off from working out. Bronchitis, if you ever had it you know, it's like breathing through a triple mask or old sock. Doctors' orders were standard 2 weeks off, no physical activity. Little did I know that it would turn into pneumonia and take me off my game for 2 years. To me that's a jail sentence. The bronchitis/pneumonia problem dragged on for 2 years. What I was left to do is live off inhalers. Seems that there is no answer for what I have. We do know that Covid has caused many of the issues with my lungs.

As of this writing it's being called LONG COVID with an Asthma side effect. Imagine someone that never smoked a day in his life with lung issues? GREAT! I sat down and read my notes. What is it I can do quickly, work muscle, keep a low heart rate and satisfy a mini workout? WITHOUT breathing too heavily! I had no lung ability, so nothing aerobic can be done. I developed a 15-minute workout for upper body it goes like this:

1. **D. Set of a DYNAMIC exercise per body part using a band or light dumbbell. (a back pull, chest press, shoulder press, triceps extension, bicep curl. 12 reps.**

2. Y. Set of the same exercises, YIELDING HOLD that I just did, this time not in full motion using band or dumbbell. This set I only hold the weight at the halfway of ISOMETRIC POSITION. 12 second hold

3. O. This time using the strap the same exercises again but strapped down in an OVERCOMING HOLD (no movement hold,) Each exercise now is pulled and held for 12 seconds with proper breathing.

3 sets that's it! 3 sets per body part. 3 days a week.
One:
Dynamic set full range.

And

Yielding set hold
Overcoming hold

I used the code 'DAYO 'on my workout
chart, it's called D.A.Y.O 911. Meaning I did
not have time or was unable to do a full
workout because of sickness or time
conflict. It was the perfect maintenance
work out until I could get back to my normal
routine. As of this writing I am working on
several other "LIMP" workouts as well.

Again, Dynamic set wait 30 seconds go, to
a Yielding hold wait 30 seconds go to
Overcoming hold. I started out doing just
one round. I found that doing it twice was
not as hard on my respiratory system. Now
whenever I have a long doctor's
appointment or am feeling sick, I do not skip

a workout. I at least do this Limp workout. This can work perfectly as well if you are running late or have a quick lunch break.

THE MIND, NERVE, MUSCLE CONNECTION

Isometric exercises can also have a positive impact on the neuromuscular connection, which refers to the communication between the nervous system and the muscles. When you perform isometric exercises, you are activating motor neurons in your muscles, which can help strengthen the connection between your nervous system and your muscles.

Here are a few ways that isometric exercises can help improve the neuro-muscular connection:

Increased motor unit recruitment: Motor units are groups of muscle fibers that are controlled by a single motor neuron. Isometric exercises can help recruit more motor units, which can help improve the connection between the nervous system and the muscles.

Improved synchronization: Isometric exercises require precise control of muscle contractions, which can help improve the synchronization between motor neurons and muscle fibers. This can improve the efficiency of muscle contractions and help prevent muscle imbalances.

Enhanced proprioception: Proprioception is the ability to sense the position, movement, and force of your body. Isometric exercises can help enhance proprioception by increasing the sensory feedback from your muscles to your nervous system. This can improve your ability to control your movements and maintain proper form during other exercises.

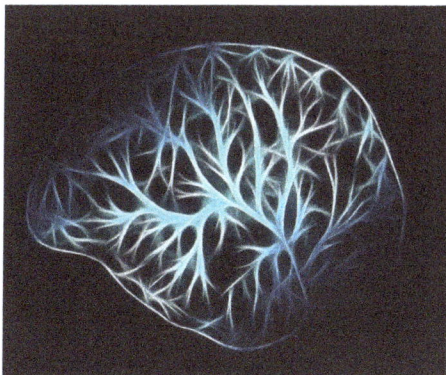

MIND MUSCLE CONNECTION

The mind-muscle connection refers to the ability to consciously contract and control a specific muscle group. Research has shown that isometric exercises can help improve the mind-muscle connection by increasing the activation of the targeted muscles and improving motor unit recruitment.

A study published in the Journal of Strength and Conditioning Research found that participants who performed isometric exercises had greater activation of the targeted muscles compared to participants who performed dynamic exercises. The researchers suggested that the increased activation was due to the isometric exercises requiring greater motor unit recruitment.

Another study published in the European Journal of Applied Physiology found that isometric exercises increased the rate of force development in the targeted muscles, which suggests improved neuromuscular coordination and activation.

NEUROMUSCULAR CONNECTION

The neuromuscular connection refers to the communication between the nervous system and the muscles. Isometric exercises can help improve the neuro-muscular connection by enhancing the synchronization between motor neurons and muscle fibers, increasing the motor unit recruitment, and enhancing proprioception.

A study published in the Journal of Applied Physiology found that isometric exercises improved the synchronization between motor neurons and muscle fibers, leading to more efficient muscle contractions. The researchers suggested that this improved synchronization was due to the isometric exercises requiring precise control of muscle contractions.

Another study published in the Journal of Neurophysiology found that isometric exercises increased the activation of motor neurons in the targeted muscles, leading to greater motor unit recruitment. The researchers suggested that this increased activation was due to the isometric exercises requiring sustained muscle contractions.

Finally, a study published in the Journal of Sport and Health Science found that isometric exercises improved proprioception by increasing the sensory feedback from the muscles to the nervous system. The researchers suggested that this enhanced proprioception was due to the isometric exercises requiring sustained muscle contractions, which increase the sensory feedback to the nervous system.

Overall, these studies suggest that isometric exercises can have a positive impact on the mind-muscle and neuromuscular connections, leading to improved muscle activation, synchronization, and proprioception.

Isometric holds have been studied for their potential to stimulate nerves and improve muscle function. Here are a few studies that have investigated the use of isometric holds for nerve stimulation:

In a study published in the Journal of Strength and Conditioning Research in 2015, researchers investigated the effects of isometric holds on the activation of the serratus anterior muscle, which is important for shoulder stability. They found that isometric holds increased muscle activation compared to other types of exercises.

Another study published in the Journal of Applied Physiology in 2010 examined the effects of isometric exercise on blood flow and neural activation in the leg muscles. The researchers found that isometric exercise increased blood flow to the muscles and improved neural activation, suggesting that isometric exercise can be an effective way to stimulate nerves and improve muscle function.

In a study published in the Journal of Rehabilitation Research and Development in 2016, researchers investigated the effects of isometric holds on muscle function in people with spinal cord injury. They found that isometric holds improved muscle function and reduced muscle spasticity in participants with spinal cord injury.

Overall, these studies suggest that isometric holds can be an effective way to stimulate nerves and improve muscle function. However, more research is needed to fully understand the mechanisms behind these effects and to decide the best use of isometric holds in clinical and rehabilitation settings.

Isometric holds involve holding a static contraction of a muscle without moving the joint. During this type of exercise, the muscle fibers are activated and generate tension, but there is no movement of the joint. Isometric holds can be performed using bodyweight or external resistance and can target specific muscle groups.

When a muscle is activated through isometric holds, the nerve fibers that innervate the muscle are also stimulated. This can lead to increased neural activation and improved muscle function over time. Isometric holds have been shown to be particularly effective for activating Type II muscle fibers, which are important for power and explosiveness.

Isometric holds may also have benefits for people with neurological conditions or injuries, such as spinal cord injury or stroke. These individuals may experience muscle weakness, spasticity, or other motor impairments. Isometric holds can be a safe and effective way to improve muscle function without risking further injury.

In addition to improving muscle function, isometric holds may also have cardiovascular benefits. Studies have shown that isometric holds can lead to increased blood flow and improved vascular function, which can be beneficial for people with cardiovascular disease or other conditions that affect blood flow.

ISOMETRIC HOLDS AND THE OVER 60 CROWD

Isometric holds, which involve contracting your muscles and holding them in a static position without movement, can be particularly beneficial for people over 60. Here are some ways that isometric holds can help this section of the population:

Improve strength and muscle mass: As we age, our muscle mass naturally decreases, leading to a loss of strength and function. Isometric holds can help to maintain and even increase muscle mass and strength, particularly in older adults who may have difficulty with traditional weightlifting exercises.

Increase bone density:

Osteoporosis, or a decrease in bone density, is a common concern for older adults. Isometric holds have been shown to help increase bone density and reduce the risk of osteoporosis.

Improve balance and stability: Falls are a major concern for older adults, and improving balance and stability can help to reduce the risk of falls. Isometric holds can help to improve balance and stability by strengthening the muscles that support the joints and improve body control.

Lower blood pressure: Isometric holds have been shown to be effective at lowering blood pressure in older adults. This is particularly important as high blood pressure can increase the risk of heart disease and stroke.

Low impact exercise: Isometric holds are low-impact exercises that can be done without putting stress on the joints. This makes them a great option for older adults who may have joint pain or limited mobility.

Some examples of isometric holds that may be suitable for older adults include wall sits, planks, and static lunges. It's important to start with lighter resistance and gradually increase the intensity and duration of your workouts as your strength and fitness level improves.

Overall, isometric holds can be a safe and effective way for older adults to improve their strength, balance, and overall physical fitness, helping them to maintain their independence and quality of life as they age.

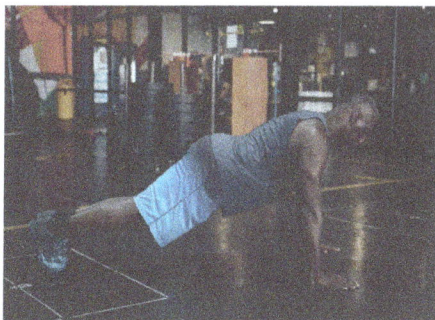

CAN ISOMETRICS ALSO HELP YOUNGER PEOPLE?

Yes, younger people can certainly receive benefits from doing isometric holds in their workout. Isometric exercises involve holding a position without movement, which can help to build strength, improve muscular endurance, and enhance overall physical fitness.

Isometric exercises can be particularly beneficial for younger people who are just starting out with their fitness journey, as they can help to build a foundation of strength and stability that can be built upon with other exercises.

Some specific benefits of isometric exercises for younger people include:

Increased strength: Isometric exercises can help to increase muscle strength, particularly in the core, back, and legs.

Improved posture: Isometric exercises can help to improve posture by strengthening the muscles that support the spine and improving overall alignment.

Reduced risk of injury: Isometric exercises can help to improve joint stability and reduce the risk of injury during other exercises or physical activities.

Increased endurance: Isometric exercises can help to improve muscular endurance, which can be helpful for sports or other physical activities that require sustained effort.

Examples of isometric exercises that younger people can incorporate into their workout routine include planks, wall sits, and static lunges. It's important to remember to start with a low intensity and gradually increase the difficulty of the exercises over time to avoid injury and maximize the benefits.

One of the benefits of isometric exercises is that they can be performed with little to no equipment, making them an accessible option for people who may not have access to a gym or other exercise equipment. Additionally, isometric exercises are low impact, which means they are less likely to cause joint pain or injury compared to exercises that involve jumping or running.

In terms of specific benefits for younger people, isometric exercises can help to improve posture, which is particularly important for those who spend a lot of time sitting or hunched over a computer or phone. Isometric exercises that target the muscles of the back and core can help to strengthen these muscles and improve alignment, which can reduce the risk of back pain and other postural issues.

Another benefit of isometric exercises is that they can help to build a foundation of strength and stability that can be built upon with other exercises. For younger people who are just starting out with their fitness journey, isometric exercises can be a good place to start to build confidence and improve overall physical fitness.

Finally, isometric exercises can be a fantastic way to improve muscular endurance, which is important for sports or other physical activities that require sustained effort. By holding a position for a period of time, isometric exercises can help to improve the ability of the muscle to continue working even when fatigued.

Overall, isometric exercises can be a valuable addition to any workout routine, particularly for younger people who are looking to improve their strength, stability, and overall physical fitness.

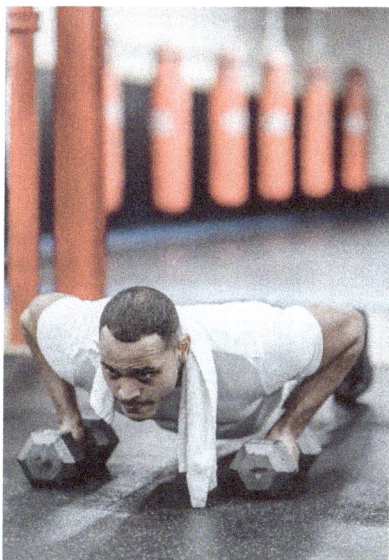

ADDING MORE INTENSITY TO ISOMETRIC HOLDS

The three position isometric holds. After you have mastered the isometric hold movement.

Incorporating isometric holds in various positions can be an effective way to work the muscle more thoroughly and promote greater strength and muscle growth.

HOLD POSITIONS

Let's take a closer look at how isometric holds in the eccentric, concentric, and isometric positions can be used to target different parts of the muscle:

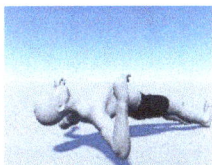

ECCENTRIC HOLD

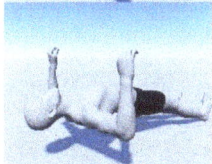

ISOMETRIC HOLD

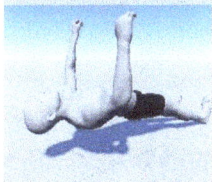

CONCENTRIC HOLD

Isometric Holds in the Eccentric
Position:

During the eccentric phase of a movement,
the muscle lengthens while under tension.
Incorporating an isometric hold in the

eccentric position can help to increase time under tension, which can lead to greater muscle damage and growth. For example, you could perform a slow eccentric lowering of a weight and hold the isometric contraction at the midpoint of the movement before lifting the weight back up.

Isometric Holds in the Isometric Position:
Incorporating isometric holds in the isometric position involves holding a static contraction without any movement. This type of hold can be used to improve muscular endurance and promote greater neuromuscular activation. For example, you could hold a plank position for an extended period of time or perform a wall sit with an isometric hold at the midpoint of the movement.

Isometric Holds in the Isometric Position:

Incorporating isometric holds in the isometric position involves holding a static contraction without any movement. The optimum hold position is about halfway through the motion. This type of hold can be used to improve muscular endurance and promote greater neuromuscular activation.

For example, you could hold a plank position for an extended period of time or perform a wall sit with an isometric hold at the midpoint of the movement. These techniques would challenge the muscles of the core and lower body, respectively, and promote greater neuromuscular activation.

It's important to note that while isometric holds can be a useful addition to your workout routine, they should be used in conjunction with a variety of other exercises and progressive overload to maximize muscle growth. Additionally, it's important to maintain proper form and alignment during the isometric holds to avoid injury.

Isometric Holds in the Concentric Position:

During the concentric phase of a movement, the muscle shortens while under tension. Incorporating an isometric hold in the concentric position can help to increase the intensity of the movement and recruit more muscle fibers. For example, you could hold a weight in the contracted position of a bicep curl before slowly lowering the weight back down.

By incorporating isometric holds in various positions, you can challenge your muscles in new ways and promote greater strength and muscle growth. It's important to note that while isometric holds can be a useful addition to your workout routine, they should be used in conjunction with a variety of other exercises and progressive overload to maximize muscle growth.

Here are some added details on how isometric holds in the eccentric, concentric, and isometric positions can be used to work the muscle better:

muscle fibers more than a regular biceps curl, as it increases the time the muscle is under tension.

WORKOUTS WHEN YOU HAVE NO TIME

A FULL BODY beginners' workout in 20 minutes?

A full body beginner isometric hold workout with one set per body part can typically be completed in around 15-20 minutes, depending on the duration of the holds and the number of exercises included in the workout.

Here is an example of a full body beginner isometric hold workout with one set per body part:

Wall sit (legs): Hold for 30-60 seconds.

Plank (core): Hold for 30-60 seconds.

Push-up hold (chest and triceps): Lower down into a push-up position and hold the halfway point for 10-30 seconds.

Superman hold (back): Lie face down and lift arms, legs, and chest off the ground and hold for 10-30 seconds.

Glute bridge hold (glutes and hamstrings): Hold a bridge position with hips lifted for 30-60 seconds.

Side plank hold (obliques): Hold the side plank position on each side for 20-30 seconds.

Isometric bicep curl (biceps): Hold a dumbbell or other weight at a 90-degree angle with your elbow and hold for 10-30 seconds.

Perform each exercise for the prescribed time and rest for 10-20 seconds between exercises. Repeat the circuit one time through. As you become more experienced, you can increase the hold times and/or add more exercises to the workout.

It's important to start with shorter hold times and gradually increase the duration over time as strength and endurance improve. And as always, please consult a qualified fitness professional before starting any new exercise program.

Isometric holds can be done in many different places, making them a convenient choice for busy people who may not have a lot of time or access to a gym. Here are some examples of where isometric holds can be done:

At home: Isometric exercises can be done in the comfort of your own home, without any equipment. You can perform wall sits, planks, static holds of the arms or legs, or other isometric exercises in a small space in your living room or bedroom.

At work: Isometric exercises can be done during breaks at work or while sitting at your desk. You can perform exercises such as squeezing a ball between your knees or holding a static hold of the arms or legs for a few seconds.

Outdoors: Isometric exercises can be done outdoors in a park or other public space. You can perform exercises such as wall sits, push-ups against a tree, or static holds of the arms or legs while standing in one place.

While traveling: Isometric exercises can be done while traveling, such as on a plane or in a hotel room. You can perform exercises such as planks, push-ups against a wall, or static holds of the arms or legs using your own body weight.

During daily activities: Isometric exercises can be incorporated into your daily activities, such as while standing in line at the grocery store or waiting for the bus. You can perform exercises such as calf raises or static holds of the arms or legs while standing in one place.

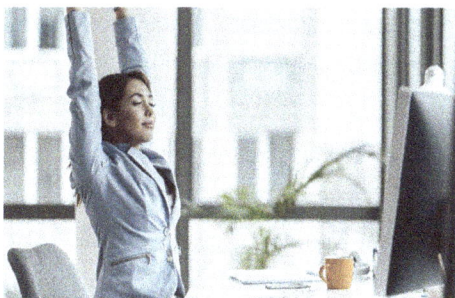

ONE SET OF THREE ANGLE HOLDS, A GREAT BEGINNING WORKOUT

Performing one set of isometric holds at eccentric, concentric, and isometric angles for 15 seconds each can be an effective way to build muscle. This type of training can help increase muscle activation, improve muscular endurance, and stimulate muscle growth.

Isometric holds at eccentric, concentric, and isometric angles each provide a different type of muscular stimulus, which can help target different muscle fibers and improve overall muscle development. Eccentric holds focus on the lengthening phase of the muscle, concentric holds focus on the shortening phase, and isometric holds focus on the static phase.

However, it's important to note that muscle growth is a complex process that depends on a variety of factors, including nutrition, rest, and overall training volume. While performing one set of isometric holds can be beneficial, it may not be enough to fully stimulate muscle growth on its own.

To maximize muscle growth, it's important to incorporate a variety of exercises and training methods into your routine, and gradually increase the volume and intensity of your training over time. This can help ensure that you are providing your muscles with the stimulus they need to grow and adapt to the demands of your training.

Building muscle is a complex process that involves a variety of factors, including nutrition, rest, and training. While isometric holds can be a useful tool for building strength and muscle, it's important to understand how they fit into an overall training program and how to use them effectively.

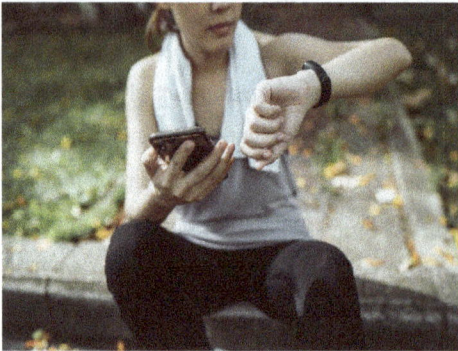

When it comes to muscle growth, there are several key factors to consider:

Progressive Overload: To stimulate muscle growth, you need to gradually increase the demands placed on your muscles over time. This can be achieved through a variety of methods, such as increasing the weight lifted, the number of sets and reps performed, or the time spent under tension. By gradually increasing the demands on your muscles, you can ensure that they are constantly adapting and growing to meet the demands of your training.

Volume: The total amount of work performed during a workout is another crucial factor in muscle growth. This includes the number of sets, reps, and exercises performed, as well as the total time spent training. While a single set of isometric holds can be beneficial, it may not provide enough volume to fully stimulate muscle growth on its own.

Nutrition: Building muscle requires a caloric surplus, which means consuming more calories than you burn each day. Additionally, you need to ensure that you are consuming enough protein to support muscle growth and recovery. A balanced diet that includes plenty of whole foods, protein, and carbohydrates can help ensure that you are providing your body with the nutrients it needs to build muscle.

Rest and Recovery: Rest and recovery are crucial for muscle growth, as this is when your muscles repair and grow stronger. Make sure to give your muscles time to recover between workouts and prioritize getting enough sleep and managing stress to support optimal recovery.

With these factors in mind, let's take a closer look at how isometric holds can be used to build muscle:

Isometric holds involve holding a static position without movement, which can improve your muscular endurance and can be useful for developing specific muscles in a targeted area. By holding a muscle contraction for an extended period, you can increase muscle activation and stimulate muscle growth.

Performing isometric holds at eccentric, concentric, and isometric angles each provides a different type of muscular stimulus, which can help target different muscle fibers and improve overall muscle development. Eccentric holds focus on the lengthening phase of the muscle, concentric holds focus on the shortening phase, and isometric holds focus on the static phase.

When incorporating isometric holds into your training program, it's important to use them in conjunction with other exercises and training methods to provide a well-rounded stimulus for your muscles. This can include compound exercises like squats, deadlifts, and bench presses, as well as isolation exercises that target specific muscle groups.

It's also important to gradually increase the volume and intensity of your isometric holds over time to ensure that your muscles are constantly adapting and growing. This can include increasing the duration of the holds, the number of sets performed, or the angle of the holds to target different muscles.

Finally, make sure to prioritize nutrition and rest to support muscle growth and recovery. This means consuming enough calories and protein to support muscle growth, as well as getting enough rest and recovery time between workouts to allow your muscles to repair and grow stronger.

THE MEDICAL USE OF ISOMETRICS

Isometric exercises are often used in medical establishments as part of a rehabilitation program for patients recovering from injuries. They can be particularly useful in the initial stages of rehabilitation when movement of the injured area is limited or contraindicated. Here are a few ways that medical establishments may use isometric exercises in post-injury rehabilitation:

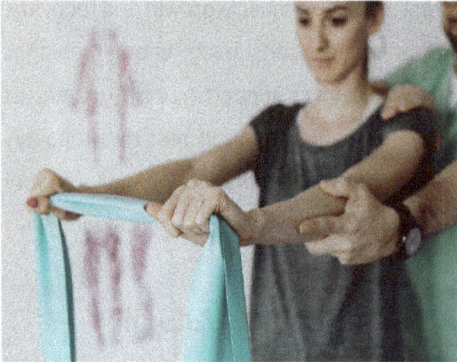

To prevent muscle atrophy: When a limb or joint is immobilized due to injury or surgery, the muscles around that area can quickly become weakened and atrophied. Isometric exercises can be used to help prevent this muscle loss by activating and strengthening the muscles without moving the joint.

To improve range of motion: Isometric exercises can also be used to help improve range of motion in a joint. By holding a muscle in a static position, the muscle fibers are activated, and the joint is gently stretched, which can help to improve flexibility and mobility.

To reduce pain and inflammation: Isometric exercises can also help to reduce pain and inflammation in the injured area. By strengthening the muscles around the injured area, isometrics can help to stabilize the joint and reduce stress on the injured tissues.

To improve overall function: Finally, isometric exercises can be used to help improve overall function and performance of the injured area. By building strength, endurance, and stability, isometrics can help patients regain their ability to perform daily activities and return to their normal level of function.

Isometric exercises can be a valuable tool in post-injury rehabilitation, helping patients to regain strength, mobility, and function in a safe and effective manner. It's important to work with a healthcare professional to develop an individualized rehabilitation program that incorporates isometric exercises in a safe and effective way.

Doctors swear by isometric exercises for their injured patients for a variety of reasons. Isometric exercises are a type of exercise that involves contracting your muscles without any movement. Unlike other types of exercises that involve movement, isometric exercises provide a way to target specific muscle groups without putting excessive stress on the injured area.

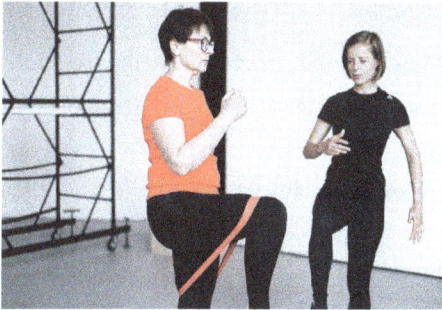

Here are some of the key reasons why doctors may recommend isometric exercises for their injured patients:

Targeted muscle strengthening: Isometric exercises can be used to target specific muscle groups that may be weakened or injured. By contracting the muscle without movement, isometric exercises can help to increase muscle strength and improve muscle function without causing further damage.

Minimal joint stress: Isometric exercises involve minimal joint stress, making them a safe and effective form of exercise for individuals with joint pain or injuries. Unlike other types of exercises that involve movement, isometric exercises do not place excessive stress on the joints, making them a good option for individuals with conditions such as arthritis or knee injuries.

Improved circulation: Isometric exercises can help to improve circulation by increasing blood flow to the muscles. This increased blood flow can help to reduce inflammation and promote healing in injured areas.

Reduced muscle wasting: Injuries can often result in muscle wasting, which is the loss of muscle mass and strength. Isometric exercises can help to prevent muscle wasting by providing a way to maintain muscle strength without movement.

Safe and easy to perform: Isometric exercises are safe and easy to perform, making them a good option for individuals who may be recovering from surgery or who have limited mobility. Isometric exercises can be performed in a variety of positions, making them accessible to individuals of all fitness levels and abilities.

THE SPRINGFIELD COLLEGE FROG ISOMETRIC EXPERIMENT

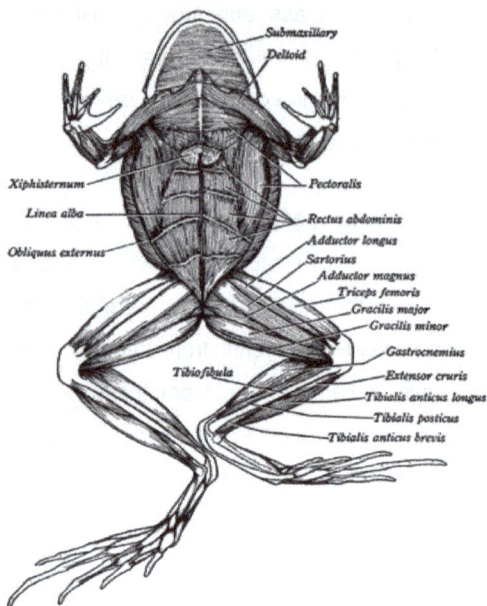

Submaxillary

Deltoid

Xiphisternum

Pectoralis

Linea alba

Rectus abdominis

Adductor longus

Obliquus externus

Sartorius

Adductor magnus

Triceps femoris

Gracilis major

Gracilis minor

Gastrocnemius

Tibiofibula

Extensor cruris

Tibialis anticus longus

Tibialis posticus

Tibialis anticus brevis

The Springfield College Frog Leg Isometric Experiment was a famous scientific experiment conducted by physiologist Henry Donaldson in the late 19th century. The experiment involved attaching electrodes to the leg muscles of a frog and measuring the force generated by the muscles when they were stimulated with an electric current.

The purpose of the experiment was to study the relationship between muscle force and muscle length, known as the length-tension relationship. Donaldson found that when the muscle was at its resting length, it generated the greatest force, and as the muscle was stretched or shortened, its force generation decreased.

The experiment is important because it helped to establish the principles of muscle physiology and the role of muscle length in force generation. It also helped to lay the groundwork for later studies on muscle mechanics and the development of exercise science.

The Springfield College Frog Leg Isometric Experiment was a significant milestone in the study of muscle physiology and contributed to our understanding of the length-tension relationship in muscle function. The experiment demonstrated that the optimal muscle length for generating the most force is at the muscle's resting length.

Subsequent research has further clarified the mechanisms underlying the length-tension relationship. For instance, studies have shown that the interaction between actin and myosin filaments within muscle fibers is affected by the length of the sarcomere, the basic unit of muscle contraction. When a sarcomere is stretched beyond its optimal length, the actin and myosin filaments have reduced overlap, and the force generated by the muscle decreases.

Additionally, research has shown that muscle architecture can affect the length-tension relationship. For instance, muscles with pennate architecture, in which fibers are arranged at an angle to the tendon, may have a different length-tension relationship than muscles with parallel architecture.

The findings from research on the length-tension relationship have practical implications for strength training and rehabilitation. For instance, strength training exercises that target muscles at their optimal length may be more effective in building muscle mass and strength. In contrast, stretching exercises that stretch muscles beyond their optimal length may reduce muscle force generation.

The Springfield College Frog Leg Isometric Experiment and research on the length-tension relationship have contributed significantly to our understanding of muscle physiology and have practical implications for exercise science and rehabilitation.

THE TOTAL BODY ISOMETRIC HOLD WORKOUT FOR THOSE THAT CAN ONLY SIT

Here is an isometric hold workout with a rope or strap for each body part while sitting down:

Equipment needed: A sturdy rope or strap (preferably with handles), a chair or bench to sit on.

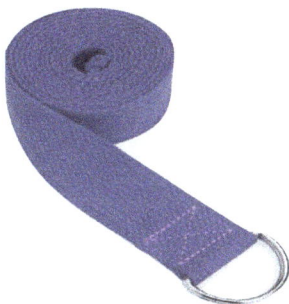

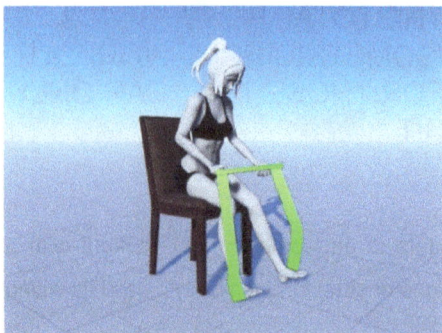

Warm-up: Before beginning the workout, it's essential to warm up your body properly. You can start with some light cardio or dynamic stretches to get your blood flowing and your muscles ready for the workout.

Chest isometric hold: Sit on the edge of a chair or bench and hold the rope with both hands. Extend your arms in front of you at shoulder height, with the rope taut. Your palms should be facing down. Hold this position for 30 seconds to 1 minute, focusing on contracting your chest muscles.

Back isometric hold: Sit on the chair or bench and hold the rope with both hands behind your back. Your palms should be facing outward, and your elbows should be bent at a 90-degree angle. Pull the rope apart, squeezing your shoulder blades together. Hold this position for 30 seconds to 1 minute, focusing on contracting your back muscles.

Shoulder isometric hold: Sit on the chair or bench and hold the rope with both hands. Your arms should be extended straight up above your head, with the rope taut. Your palms should be facing each other. Hold this position for 30 seconds to 1 minute, focusing on contracting your shoulder muscles.

Bicep isometric hold: Sit on the chair or bench and hold the rope with one hand. Your arm should be extended straight down at your side, with the rope taut. Your palm should be facing up. Curl the rope up towards your shoulder, contracting your bicep muscle. Hold this position for 30 seconds to 1 minute, focusing on contracting your bicep muscle.

Triceps isometric hold: Sit on the chair or bench and hold the rope with one hand behind your head. Your elbow should be bent, and your forearm should be pointing down at your back. Pull the rope up towards the ceiling, contracting your triceps muscle. Hold this position for 30 seconds to 1 minute, focusing on contracting your triceps muscle.

Abdominal isometric hold: Sit on the chair or bench and hold the rope with both hands. Your arms should be extended straight out in front of you at shoulder height, with the rope taut. Lean back slightly and engage your core muscles. Hold this position for 30 seconds to 1 minute, focusing on contracting your abdominal muscles.

Quadricep isometric hold: Sit on the chair or bench and tie the rope around one ankle. Extend your leg out in front of you, with the rope taut. Your other foot should be flat on the ground. Push your foot forward into the rope, contracting your quadricep muscle. Hold this position for 30 seconds to 1 minute, focusing on contracting your quadricep muscle.

Hamstring isometric hold: Sit on the chair or bench and tie the rope around one ankle. Extend your leg out in front of you, with the rope taut. Your other foot should be flat on the ground. Pull your foot back towards your body, contracting your hamstring muscle. Hold this position for 30 seconds to 1 minute, focusing on contracting your hamstring muscle.

Cool-down: After completing the workout, it's important to cool down properly. You can do some light static stretches to help your muscles recover and prevent soreness.

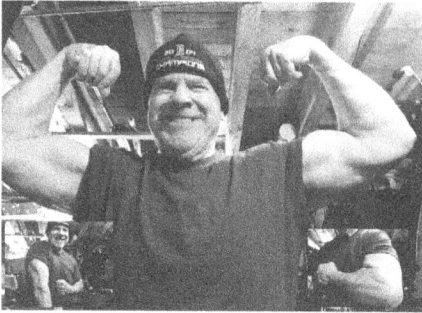

Note: It's important to listen to your body during this workout and not overdo it. Start with shorter holds and work your way up to longer holds as you become more comfortable with the exercises.

Thank You for taking the time to read this book. We have found this to be a VERY useful exercise program especially when you are limited on time, are recovering from injury or just don't know where to start. You can find more information on our blog as well.

www.isoquickstrength.blogspot.com

or

www.isoquickstrength.com

ISO QUICK

STRENGTH

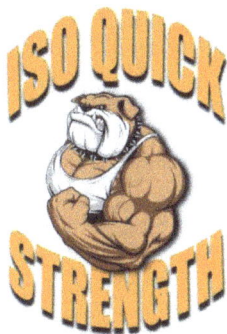

EVERYTHING ISOMETRIC

Customized HYBRID Program

HYSOMETRICS

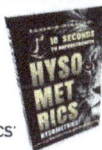

LOOK FOR OUR BOOK 'HYSOMETRICS'

www.ingramcontent.com/pod-product-compliance
Lightning Source LLC
Chambersburg PA
CBHW051717020426
42333CB00014B/1023